Biology of Orthodontic Tooth Movement

Bhavna Shroff
Editor

Biology of Orthodontic Tooth Movement

Current Concepts and Applications in Orthodontic Practice

Springer

Editor
Bhavna Shroff
Department of Orthodontics
VCU School of Dentistry
Richmond, Virginia
USA

ISBN 978-3-319-26607-7 ISBN 978-3-319-26609-1 (eBook)
DOI 10.1007/978-3-319-26609-1

Library of Congress Control Number: 2016942276

Printed on acid-free paper

This Springer imprint is published by Springer Nature
The registered company is Springer International Publishing AG Switzerland

Preface

Biology has always been an integral part of orthodontics. The biological processes behind the orthodontic movement of teeth have been a source of scientific curiosity since the early parts of the twentieth century, and visionaries like C. Sandstedt, A. Oppenheim, B. Orban, and A. H. Ketcham established a long-lasting relationship between the two fields. The controversies about the use of light or heavy forces during orthodontic tooth movement and the observations of the biological effects of such forces on teeth, periodontal ligament, and supporting bone have gradually shifted to a more profound and better understanding of the mechanisms involved in the remodeling of those tissues and cellular event associated with it. It is with gratitude that we can recognize pioneers like Reitan, Davidovitch, and Per Rygh as major contributors, who introduced new ways to study this field.

In more recent years, the interest in the biology of tooth movement has shifted to a different set of priorities. As a specialty, we started a conversation about how to use our fundamental understanding of orthodontic tooth movement to accelerate the movement of teeth through the bone. We are also using this knowledge to attempt to control, minimize, and also predict the occurrence of iatrogenic effects and, ultimately, to bring to our patients a better experience during their treatment.

This book is primarily the work of people who are passionate about the biology of orthodontic tooth movement. They have dedicated a life time to the study and the understanding of how teeth move when we treat our patients. They have been inspired by their mentors who instilled in them this scientific curiosity and the power to ask the questions discussed in this book. This book is not only an account of our current knowledge of this field but also an opportunity to look into the future and see the possibilities that will be available to the clinician to improve the treatment of the people that we serve.

As to me, I am grateful to my family, my teachers, and mentors. They made me who I am today, and they gave me the greatest gifts of all, the curiosity to ask questions and the passion for what I do. I wish to dedicate this book to Professor Jean-Claude Kaqueler who introduced me to research and electron microscopy, Dr. Charles J. Burstone who made me love orthodontics, and to Dr. Ravindra Nanda for his unwavering support along this extraordinary journey.

You have my eternal gratitude.

Richmond, VA, USA

Bhavna Shroff

Contents

Role of Alveolar Bone in Mediating Orthodontic Tooth Movement and Relapse

1

Imad Maleeh, Jennifer Robinson, and Sunil Wadhwa

Abstract

In this chapter, we present a unique perspective on biological tooth movement, one that describes the adaptive nature of the alveolar bone in response to mechanical loading. We provide a new foundation to the classical "pressure-tension" theory of orthodontic tooth movement. The chapter describes the individual roles of the cell types of bone (osteoblasts, osteoclasts, osteocytes, osteoprogenitor cells, and bone lining cells) in response to tooth movement, largely focusing on the mechanosensing osteocytes. Also discussed are methods that possibly increase the rate of orthodontic tooth movement as well as the plausible role that osteocytes may have in mediating relapse. Finally, we conclude with an "overall model of tooth movement and relapse." This chapter attempts to present an upstream mechanism to the traditional "pressure-tension" theory based on the most recent evidence.

German anatomist and surgeon Julius Wolff was the first to describe the adaptive nature of bone in response to the mechanical loads under which it is placed. Bone mass and architecture are determined primarily by loading patterns (magnitude and direction), which cause the bone trabeculae and cortex to remodel accordingly [1].

I. Maleeh, DDS • S. Wadhwa, DDS, PhD (✉)
Division of Orthodontics, Columbia University College of Dental Medicine,
622 W. 168th Street, VC 9-219, New York, NY 10032, USA
e-mail: im2313@cumc.columbia.edu; Sw2680@cumc.columbia.edu

J. Robinson, PhD
Division of Orthodontics, Columbia University College of Dental Medicine,
622 W. 168th Street, VC 9-219, New York, NY 10032, USA

Department of Biomedical Engineering, Columbia University, New York, NY, USA
e-mail: Jlr2228@columbia.edu

B. Shroff (ed.), *Biology of Orthodontic Tooth Movement*,
DOI 10.1007/978-3-319-26609-1_1

Increases in bone mass result from increased mechanical strains, such as physical activity [2]. On the other hand, decreased strain magnitude from prolonged bed rest leads to bone loss [3]. Similar to long bones, the alveolar bone that houses the dentition acclimates to changes in occlusal loading. However, the mechanisms in which occlusal forces are transferred to the alveolar bone have the added complexity of an intervening medium, the periodontal ligament (PDL). Orthodontic tooth movement (OTM) is based on the aforementioned biological principle; intermittent or continuous forces are applied to teeth, changing the mechanical loading of the system and subsequently eliciting a cellular response that leads to bone adaptation in a new functional environment. Many theories have been described in the literature with the attempt to elucidate the mechanisms involved in biological tooth movement. Most in vivo studies have concentrated on changes occurring within the PDL; however, more recent proposals have focused on the response of the alveolar bone [4]. In this chapter, we will concentrate on the recent studies showing that tooth movement may be more heavily dictated by the alveolar bone as opposed to the PDL.

1.1 Cell Types Involved in OTM

There are five types of cells identified in the alveolar bone that respond to orthodontic tooth movement: osteoblasts, osteoclasts, osteocytes, osteoprogenitor cells, and bone lining cells [5]. Osteoblasts are of mesenchymal origin and are primarily the bone-forming cells. Osteoblasts synthesize and secrete the extracellular matrix of bone, including type 1 collagen. Several factors have been shown to influence the development of osteoblasts from mesenchymal progenitor cells in the PDL. The factors include bone morphogenetic proteins (BMPs), transforming growth factor (TGF-βI and II), insulin-like growth factor (IGF-I and II), platelet-derived growth factor (PDGF), and fibroblast growth factor (FGF) [6]. In addition to their bone-forming capabilities, osteoblasts lining the bony socket are now believed to respond directly to strain from orthodontic tooth movement through a process known as mechanotransduction [7].

The second type of cells are the osteoclasts, which are derived from hematopoietic stem cells. Osteoclasts are responsible for the bone resorption necessary for tooth movement. Soluble factors such as colony-stimulating factor (CSF), receptor activator of nuclear factor-kappa B ligand (RANKL), osteoprotegerin (OPG), and bone morphogenic proteins (BMPs) regulate osteoclast differentiation [8–10]. These factors are produced by osteocytes found in the alveolar bone and osteoblasts found in the PDL [11]. CSF as well as RANKL and its receptor RANK promote differentiation of osteoclasts. OPG inhibits differentiation by acting as a decoy receptor for RANKL, thus inhibiting its binding to RANK [12].

The third type of cell is the osteocyte, which is believed to be a terminally differentiated osteoblast that is surrounded by the bone matrix and whose function is primarily proprioceptive and responsive [13]. Osteocytes communicate with neighboring osteocytes and osteoblasts on the bone surface via long cytoplasmic extensions, in which direct exchange of ions occurs through connections called gap junctions. The osteocytes reside within the bone in a space called a lacuna, and their cytoplasmic processes are housed within small canals called canaliculi. They are thought to be the mechanosensory cells of bone that play a pivotal role in functional adaptation to changing loading patterns [14].

The fourth cell type is the bone lining cell, which is also thought to be a terminally differentiated osteoblast. Lining cells are involved in bone protection and maintenance of bone fluids [15]. They may also be involved in the propagation of the activation signal that initiates bone resorption and bone remodeling [15]. Lastly, osteoprogenitor cells are the stem cell population tasked with generating osteoblasts and are situated in the vicinity of blood vessels of the PDL [16].

Orthodontic tooth movement occurs as a result of a complex sequence of events that involves cell-cell and cell-matrix interactions as well as a conglomeration of systemic hormones, cytokines, and growth factors. Recent research has pointed to osteocytes and osteoblasts lining the alveolar within the PDL as key cells regulating orthodontic tooth movement.

1.2 Osteocytes May Be Responsible for Mediating Orthodontic Tooth Movement Resorption

Orthodontic tooth movement was historically described by the "pressure-tension theory." This theory was first developed through classic histologic studies and led researchers to postulate that within the bony socket, "pressure" and "tension" sides were generated after force application [17–19]. The theory hypothesizes the side that the tooth is moving toward causes pressure/compression of the PDL (also named the "compression" side). Compression of the PDL is then believed to cause constriction of the blood vessels within the PDL causing a lack of nutrient flow and subsequent hyalinization and cell death. Osteoclasts from within the PDL (frontal resorption) or from the adjacent bone marrow (undermining resorption) invade the area and resorb the hyalinized PDL and adjacent alveolar bone causing the tooth to move [20]. On the contralateral side of the socket, namely, the "tension side," PDL fibers are stretched leading to stimulation of bone deposition. This theory simplifies tooth movement to a 2-dimensional process, namely, the mesial and distal ends. More recently, studies have described resorptive patches localized more lingually or buccally of the moving teeth. This is likely a consequence of irregularities in the periodontal and bone morphology, which illuminates the 3-dimensional nature of tooth movement [21]. Due to the presence of the PDL fibers between the tooth and the bone, the terminology of this theory is confounding. The "pressure or compression" side suggests loading of the bone, when in actuality the PDL fibers develop laxity and thus are unloaded or could be under tension [22]. On the "tension" side, stretched PDL fibers are seen, causing the loading of bone and bony matrix deposition. For the sake of clarity, we will therefore eliminate the use of compression and tension and refer to the compression side as the direction in which the tooth is moving and tension as the direction opposite to the direction of tooth movement (Fig. 1.1).

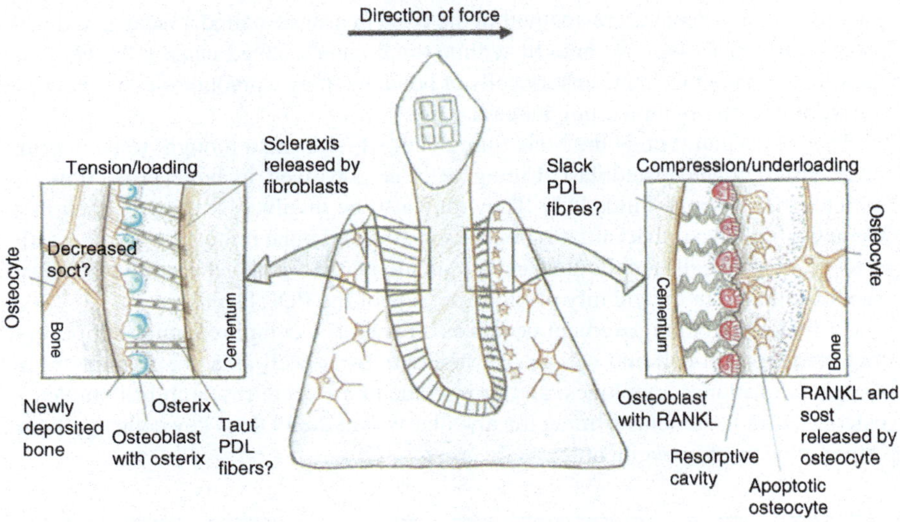

Fig. 1.1 Model of orthodontic tooth movement. On the direction the tooth is moving, orthodontic force causes an increase in apoptotic osteocytes and increase in the production of RankL. On the side opposite to the direction of tooth movement, orthodontic force causes an increase in the production of scleraxis in PDL fibroblasts and an increase in osterix in the PDL alveolar lining cells

In the direction in which the tooth is moving, osteoclasts are required to resorb the alveolar bone in order to allow for orthodontic tooth movement. The exact mechanism for the recruitment of the osteoclasts remains unknown. However, recent evidence points to osteocytes controlling alveolar bone resorption. Evidence that osteocytes are responsible for osteoclast bone resorption during orthodontic tooth movement comes from a study in transgenic mice in which the osteocytes were ablated. These mice express the receptor for diphtheria toxin on the cell surfaces of osteocytes. Therefore, an injection of diphtheria toxin caused osteocyte cell death. It was found that orthodontic tooth movement in the later phase was significantly reduced in transgenic mice with osteocyte cell death. Further, the number of osteoclasts and the quantity of eroded bone surface were significantly reduced in the transgenic mice injected with diphtheria toxin than in control mice [23].

It is established that osteocytes are the mechanosensing cells within the bone [24]. Osteocytes form a lacunar-canalicular network that allows their communication with other osteocyte, osteoblast, and osteoclast progenitors [24]. Mechanical loading-induced fluid flow through the lacunar-canalicular network provides nutrients to osteocytes and the upregulation of anabolic factors [25]. In contrast, loss of loading causes a decrease in fluid flow and increased osteocyte apoptosis. Birte Melsen was one of the first to posit that the resorption seen in orthodontic tooth movement is associated with alveolar bone underloading [26]. Meikle followed her study and used Frost's principle of a "mechanostat" to help support her findings. The fundamental idea of this principle is that for each bone in the skeleton, there is a functional adapted state within the boundaries of which normal bone mass is maintained [27]. It was found that the use of an orthodontic appliance (cross-arch spring bonded to the teeth) changes the dynamics of the stimuli received by the bone and has a negative effect on bone mass. A bonded appliance, whether active or passive, was sufficient to alter the loading dynamics of the teeth, shielding some areas of bone from stress and leading to bone loss and osteopenia [4]. This osteopenia resulted from stress shielding of the interradicular bone by the appliance and a consequent reduction in occlusal loading below the critical threshold required for maintaining normal osseous architecture.

Osteocytes cause increased bone resorption during an underloading state by releasing RANKL and undergoing apoptosis. RANKL is the key molecule involved in the maturation of osteoclasts. In bone, osteocytes are the major producers of RANKL and cause an increase in osteoclastogenesis by releasing soluble RANKL through the lacunar-canalicular network. This promotes its interaction with osteoclast precursors to stimulate their differentiation and activation [28]. Therefore, the increase in orthodontic tooth movement-induced RANKL expression may result from osteocytes within the alveolar bone. This may explain why tooth movement in mice in which the osteocytes are ablated has a decrease in osteoclastic bone resorption [23].

We and others have found that orthodontic tooth movement causes a significant increase in osteocyte apoptosis within 1 or 2 days [29]. We also found that osteoclast recruitment occurred after 72 h and was particularly evident at day 7 after the initiation of orthodontic force. This suggests that osteoclastogenesis commences later than the peak of osteocyte apoptosis, suggesting that it is a downstream effect [29]. Apoptotic osteocytic bodies have been shown to release potent factors that cause an increase in osteoclasts [30–32]. It may seem paradoxical that osteocyte apoptosis causes an increase in osteoclast resorption, whereas osteocyte ablation causes an inhibition of osteoclast bone resorption. These confounding results may be explained by the type of cell death and/or the amount of cell death. In osteocyte ablation, it is presumed that osteocyte cell death occurs via necrosis [33], which may cause a differential response for osteoclastogenesis as compared to osteocyte apoptosis. Further it may also be possible that cell death of a finite number of osteocytes causes bone resorption, whereas cell death of all the alveolar bone osteocytes causes inhibition of osteoclast resorption. Future studies on the role of OTM-induced osteocyte apoptosis on osteoclast resorption are needed in order to clarify this issue.

1.3 Osteoblast Progenitors Within the PDL and Alveolar Bone Lining Cells Mediate New Bone Formation

The periodontal ligament is composed of alveolar bone lining osteoblastic cells and fibroblastic PDL cells. In the direction opposite to which the tooth is moving, upregulation of osterix within the alveolar bone lining cells and scleraxis within the periodontal fibroblasts occurs [34]. Osterix is an osteoblast differentiation factor, and its upregulation is associated with new bone formation. In mice that are deficient in osterix, no bone formation occurs [35]. In contrast, scleraxis upregulation is associated with tendon formation and has been shown to cause downregulation of osteoblast differentiation [34]. Therefore, the upregulation of scleraxis with the PDL fibroblasts prevents its calcification and maintains its patency, whereas upregulation of osterix on the alveolar bone lining osteoblasts causes deposition of new bone on its surface. We have also found the upregulation of the bone maturation marker bone sialoprotein (BSP) in alveolar bone lining cells on the side opposite the direction of tooth movement [36]. BSP is also associated with matrix calcification [37]. Taken together, the results suggest that the OTM process, on the side opposite the direction of tooth movement, causes osteoblast differentiation of the osteoblast lining cells of the periodontal ligament.

However, whether the increase in bone formation is due to changes in the mechanical loading environment of the osteoblast lining cells within the PDL or instead caused by soluble factors released by osteocytes within the alveolar bone remains unknown. Evidence that it may be from osteocytes comes from a classical study by Heller and Nanda in which they gave a lathrytic agent that caused disruption of the collagen fibers within the PDL. In this study, they found that OTM caused an increase in new bone formation on the side opposite of tooth movement in animals treated with control and the lathrytic agent. From these results, the authors concluded that the PDL-induced fiber tension on the alveolar osteoblast lining cells may not be absolutely necessary to stimulate bone formation during OTM. Instead distortion of the alveolus bone related to force application may be a more important factor initiating the new bone formation [38]. It has also been shown that osteocyte production of sclerostin was reduced on the side opposite to the tooth movement [39]. Sclerostin is mainly produced by osteocytes and inhibits the Wnt signaling pathway, and its downregulation is associated with new bone formation [40]. Therefore, the new bone formation seen on the side opposite to which the tooth is moving may be due to osteocytic decrease in soluble Sost, which is a known Wnt signaling inhibitor. The net effect is an increase in Wnt signaling within the alveolar bone lining cells, an increase in osterix and BSP expression, and new bone formation. Future studies examining new bone formation on the side opposite to the tooth movement in transgenic mice with alteration in Sost signaling are needed to clarify this issue.

1.4 Methods to Increase the Rate of Orthodontic Tooth Movement

Several approaches to accelerate orthodontic tooth movement by altering bone biology have been proposed. Currently, two main methods exist for accelerating tooth movement by altering bone biology: (1) induced local bone damage, i.e., corticotomy-assisted orthodontics, piezocision-aided orthodontics, and corticision, and (2) mechanical loading-induced remodeling, i.e., vibration. Local bone damage-assisted OTM is performed by perforating the cortical bone or by making local incisions around the cortical bone. The biological basis for this modality is that local bone damage (i.e., microcracks) has been shown to cause an increase in osteoclast activity and bone remodeling [41]. Case reports in the literature and small clinical trials have demonstrated a modest increase in the rate of initial OTM by these methods [42–44]. However, this effect was not seen in the long term. In addition, we have performed a recent study in which we evaluated the effect of applied force with and without corticision. We found no differences in the rate of tooth movement and osteoclastic bone resorption between animals that received the corticision procedure versus those who did not in a rat model [45]. Taken together, the results suggest that corticotomy, corticision, and/or piezocision results in a modest change in the rate of initial orthodontic tooth movement. This may be due to the fact that the resorption seen in the later phases in OTM is due to underloading of osteocytes in the alveolar bone, which is not affected by local bone damage procedures. In support, osteocyte ablation caused a decrease only in the later phases of tooth movement [23]. Also, OTM-associated microcracks are seen in both directions in which the tooth is moving and not limited only to the resorption side [46]. The early increase in OTM seen in bone damage-associated tooth movement may be associated with the fact that osteoclast recruitment does not occur immediately after the application of orthodontic force, but rather 3–7 days later [29]. Therefore, the increase in the initial phase of tooth movement by local bone damage may be due to an earlier recruitment of osteoclasts.

Recently, the use of resonance vibration has been developed as a new treatment modality for accelerating tooth movement. This idea contradicts the traditional use of vibration for increasing bone mass. Whole body vibration has demonstrated significant increases in bone mineral density and structure due to the mechanosensory functions of osteocytes [24, 47, 48]. Therefore, the anabolic effect provided by vibration would theoretically inhibit tooth movement by preventing OTM-associated osteocyte underloading. In fact, Kalajzic et al. showed that vibration in rats decreased the rate of tooth movement [49]. Moreover, Woodhouse et al. found no evidence that supplemental vibration force increased the rate of initial tooth alignment or reduced the time required to achieve complete alignment [50]. Taken together, the results suggest that the effects of vibration on accelerating orthodontic tooth movement are not due to a biological response. On the contrary, the effects may have more to do with frictional sliding forces.

1.5 Retention

One of the most pressing issues in orthodontic treatment is tooth relapse. Relapse is defined as the tendency of teeth to return toward their pretreatment positions [51]. Specifically, its occurrence renders treatment failure for both the orthodontist and the patient. Instability of orthodontically aligned teeth occurs to some extent in almost every patient [52]. The etiologic factors that drive relapse are still unclear; however, several causes have been proposed. Relapse is believed to be complex and multifactorial, including factors such as inter-canine width [53], mandibular growth rotation [54], facial growth [55, 56], third molar eruption [57], influence of stretched gingival and connective tissue fibers [58–62], treatment modalities [63], uncooperative patients, imbalance in muscle and soft tissue pressure [64, 65], arch dimensions [66], and ongoing bone turnover [67]. However, it is now becoming clear that orthodontic tooth movement and relapse occur via the same biological mechanisms, regardless of the initial force applied.

Similar to orthodontic tooth movement, orthodontic relapse is associated with increased osteoclast activity and apoptosis on the side in which the tooth is moving [68]. One of the big differences between OTM and relapse is that relapse is associated with an increase in alveolar bone density, whereas OTM is associated with a decrease. For example, Franzen et al. demonstrated that after appliance removal, tissue mineral density and bone volume percentage gradually increased as the course of relapse progressed, attaining control levels after 3 days [69]. The return of bone density back to the levels of pre-orthodontic tooth movement during relapse leads one to speculate that changes in osteocyte mechanical loading environment may also mediate relapse. This is consistent with the findings of increased osteoclasts and an increase in apoptosis during orthodontic relapse. However, studies with osteocyte ablation and relapse are needed in order to further investigate this hypothesis.

1.6 Overall Model of Tooth Movement and Relapse

In our working model, we posit that when an orthodontic force is applied to the teeth, it causes a change in the mechanical loading environment of the osteocytes within the adjacent alveolar bone. In the direction in which the tooth is moving, there is an underloading state causing osteocytes to release factors (RANKL) and undergo apoptosis, both of which promote osteoclastic bone resorption. On the side opposite to direction of tooth movement, osteocytes undergo an increased loading response causing them to inhibit their release of Sost which promotes new bone formation from osteoblasts lining the alveolar bone. The net effect of OTM is an overall reduction in alveolar bone density due to increased bone resorption relative to new bone formation.

After the cessation of OTM and removal of the forces applied to alveolar bone from braces, a portion of the alveolar bone may be in an underloading state. This causes osteocytes to release RANKL and undergo apoptosis causing bone and tooth remodeling. The net effect is the return of alveolar bone density baseline levels and repositioning of the teeth close to their original position. Efforts to accelerate the rate of orthodontic tooth movement may occur by further reducing the underloading-induced bone remodeling state. Furthermore, retention strategies should be aimed at increasing alveolar bone density after the cessation of orthodontic tooth movement. Reducing the underloading remodeling state to accelerate orthodontic tooth movement is difficult to achieve. This may explain the modest effects experienced over the past century. On the other hand, trying to increase bone density after the cessation of tooth movement to prevent relapse may be easier to achieve. For example, externally applied vibration in conjunction with retainer wear may further enhance tooth stability [70].

Conclusion

Traditionally, orthodontic tooth movement was believed to occur by causing necrosis of the PDL, causing the recruitment of osteoclasts and subsequent resorption and tooth movement. However, recent studies have now suggested that tooth movement may be due to alterations in the mechanical loading state of alveolar bone osteocytes. On the side in which the tooth is moving, there may be an underloading state causing osteocytes to release RANKL which increases bone resorption. On the other side, an increased loading state in which the osteocytes decrease their release of Sost resulting in an increase in bone formation may exist. Because these two theories are not mutually exclusive, it is possible that a combination of the two is occurring. It is now evident that the traditional idea that OTM solely occurs by necrosis and hyalinization of the PDL is a misconception.

References

1. Frost HM. Wolff's Law and bone's structural adaptations to mechanical usage: an overview for clinicians. Angle Orthod. 1994;64:175–88.
2. Nilsson BE, Westlin NE. Bone density in athletes. Clin Orthop Relat Res. 1971;77:179–82.
3. Donaldson CL, et al. Effects of prolonged bed rest on bone mineral. Metabolism. 1970;19:1071–84.
4. Milne TJ, et al. Induction of osteopenia during experimental tooth movement in the rat: alveolar bone remodeling and the mechanostat theory. Eur J Orthod. 2009;31:221–31.
5. Patil AK, et al. Understanding the advances in biology of orthodontic tooth movement for improved ortho-perio interdisciplinary approach. J Indian Soc Perio. 2013;17:309–18.
6. Harada S, Rodan GA. Control of osteoblast function and regulation of bone mass. Nature. 2003;423:349–55.
7. Sandy JR, et al. Recent advances in understanding mechanically induced bone remodeling and their relevance to orthodontic theory and practice. Am J Orthod Dentofacial Orthop. 1993;103:212–22.
8. Nomura S, Takano-Yamamoto T. Molecular events caused by mechanical stress in bone. Matrix Biol. 2000;19:91–6.
9. Zhao S, et al. MLO-Y4 osteocyte-like cells support osteoclast formation and activation. J Bone Miner Res. 2002;17:2068–79.
10. Kurata K, et al. Bone marrow cell differentiation induced by mechanically damaged osteocytes in 3D gel-embedded culture. J Bone Miner Res. 2006;21:616–25.
11. Oshiro T, et al. Osteoclast induction in periodontal tissue during experimental movement of incisors in osteoprotegerin-deficient mice. Anat Rec. 2002;266:218–25.
12. Theoleyre S, et al. The molecular triad OPG/RANK/RANKL: involvement in the orchestration of pathophysiological bone remodeling. Cytokine Growth F R. 2004;15:457–75.
13. Weinbaum S, et al. A model for the excitation of osteocytes by mechanical loading-induced bone fluid shear stresses. J Biomech. 1994;27:339–60.
14. Aarden EM, et al. Function of osteocytes in bone. J Cell Biochem. 1994;55(3):287–99.

15. Miller SC, et al. Bone lining cells: structure and function. Scanning Microsc. 1989;3:953–60.
16. Agata H, et al. Effective bone engineering with periosteum-derived cells. J Dent Res. 2007;86:79–83.
17. Sandstedt C. Einige beitrage zur theorie der zahnregulierung. Nord Tandlaeg Tidskr. 1904;5:236–56.
18. Oppenheim A. Tissue changes, particularly of the bone, incident to tooth movement. Am J Orthod. 1911;3:57–67.
19. Schwarz AM. Tissue changes incident to orthodontic tooth movement. Int J Orthod. 1932;18:331–52.
20. Reitan K. Some factors determining the evaluation of force in orthodontics. Am J Orthod. 1957;43:32–45.
21. Bohl MV, et al. Focal hyalinization during experimental tooth movement in beagle dogs. Am J Orthod Dentofacial Orthop. 2004;125:615–23.
22. Jiang F, et al. Mechanical environment change in root, periodontal ligament, and alveolar bone in response to two canine retraction treatment strategies. Orthod Craniofac Res. 2015;18 Suppl 1:29–38.
23. Matsumoto T, et al. The role of osteocytes in bone resorption during orthodontic tooth movement. J Dent Res. 2013;92(4):340–5.
24. Bonewald LF. The amazing osteocyte. J Bone Miner Res. 2011;26(2):229–38.
25. Qin YX, Hu M. Mechanotransduction in musculoskeletal tissue regeneration: effects of fluid flow, loading, and cellular-molecular pathways. Biomed Res Int. 2014;863421(12).
26. Melsen B. Tissue reaction to orthodontic tooth movement–a new paradigm. Eur J Orthod. 2001;23(6):671–81.
27. Frost HM. Bone 'mass' and the 'mechanostat': a proposal. Anat Rec. 1987;219:1–9.
28. Nakashima T, et al. Evidence for osteocyte regulation of bone homeostasis through RANKL expression. Nat Med. 2011;17(10):1231–4.
29. Moin S, et al. Osteocyte death during orthodontic tooth movement in mice. Angle Orthod. 2014;84(6):1086–92.
30. Mori S, Burr DB. Increased intracortical remodeling following fatigue damage. Bone. 1993;14:103–9.
31. Taylor D, Lee TC. Microdamage and mechanical behavior: predicting failure and remodeling in compact bone. J Anat. 2003;203:203–11.
32. Noble B. Microdamage and apoptosis. Eur J Morphol. 2005;42:91–8.
33. Komori T. Mouse models for the evaluation of osteocyte functions. J Bone Metab. 2014;21(1):55–60.
34. Takimoto A, et al. Scleraxis and osterix antagonistically regulate tensile force-responsive remodeling of the periodontal ligament and alveolar bone. Development. 2015;142(4):787–96.
35. Sinha KM, Zhou X. Genetic and molecular control of osterix in skeletal formation. J Cell Biochem. 2013;114(5):975–84.
36. Olson C, et al. Orthodontic tooth movement causes decreased promoter expression of collagen type 1, bone sialoprotein and alpha-smooth muscle actin in the periodontal ligament. Orthod Craniofac Res. 2012;15(1):52–61.
37. Kruger TE, Miller AH, Wang J. Collagen scaffolds in bone sialoprotein-mediated bone regeneration. Scientific World J. 2013;812718(6).
38. Heller IJ, Nanda R. Effect of metabolic alteration of periodontal fibers on orthodontic tooth movement. An experimental study. Am J Orthod. 1979;75(3):239–58.
39. Nishiyama Y, et al. Changes in the spatial distribution of sclerostin in the osteocytic lacuno-canalicular system in alveolar bone due to orthodontic forces, as detected on multimodal confocal fluorescence imaging analyses. Arch Oral Biol. 2015;60(1):45–54.
40. Compton JT, Lee FY. A review of osteocyte function and the emerging importance of sclerostin. J Bone Joint Surg Am. 2014;96(19):1659–68.

41. Huang H, et al. Accelerated orthodontic tooth movement: molecular mechanisms. Am J Orthod Dentofacial Orthop. 2014;146:620–32.
42. Dibart S, et al. Piezocision: a minimally invasive, periodontally accelerated orthodontic tooth movement procedure. Compend Contin Educ Dent. 2009;30:342–4, 46, 48–50.
43. Dibart S, et al. Rapid treatment of class II malocclusion with piezocision: two case reports. Int J Periodontics Restorative Dent. 2010;30:487–93.
44. Keser EL, Dibart S. Piezocision-assisted Invisalign treatment. Compend Contin Educ Dent. 2011;32:46–8, 50–51.
45. Murphy CA, et al. Effect of corticision and different force magnitudes on orthodontic tooth movement in a rat model. Am J Orthod Dentofacial Orthop. 2014;146(1):55–66.
46. Prager TM, et al. Microdamage in the alveolar process of rat maxillae after orthodontic tooth movement. J Orofac Orthop. 2015;76(1):41–50.
47. Rubin C, et al. Low mechanical signals strengthen long bones. Nature. 2001;412:603–4.
48. Prisby RD, et al. Effects of whole body vibration on the skeleton and other organ systems in man and animal models: what we know and what we need to know. Ageing Res Rev. 2008;7:319–29.
49. Kalajzic Z, et al. Effect of cyclical forces on the periodontal ligament and alveolar bone remodeling during orthodontic tooth movement. Angle Orthod. 2014;84(2):297–303.
50. Woodhouse NR, et al. Supplemental vibrational force during orthodontic alignment: a randomized trial. J Dent Res. 2015;94:682–9.
51. Dyer KC, et al. Relapse revisited- again. Am J Orthod Dentofacial Orthop. 2012;142:221–7.
52. Joondeph DR. Retention and relapse. In: Graber TM, Vanarsdall RL, Vig KWL, editors. Orthodontics: Current Principles and Techniques. St Louis: Elsevier Mosby; 2005. p. 1123–51.
53. Rossouw PE, et al. A longitudinal evaluation of the anterior border of the dentition. Am J Orthod Dentofacial Orthop. 1993;104:146–52.
54. Fudalej P, et al. Mandibular growth rotation effects on postretention stability of mandibular incisor alignment. Angle Orthod. 2007;77:199–205.
55. Driscoll-Gilliland J, et al. An evaluation of growth and stability in untreated and treated subjects. Am J Orthod Dentofac Orthop. 2001;120:588–97.
56. Sinclair PM, et al. Maturation of untreated normal occlusions. Am J Orthod. 1983;83:114–23.
57. Harradine NW, et al. The effect of extraction of third molars on late lower incisor crowding: a randomized controlled trial. Br J Orthod. 1998;25:117–22.
58. Edwards JG. A long-term prospective evaluation of the circumferential supracrestal fiberotomy in alleviating orthodontic relapse. Am J Orthod Dentofacial Orthop. 1988;93:380–7.
59. Bergstrom K, et al. The effect of superior labial frenectomy in cases with midline diastema. Am J Orthod. 1973;63:633–8.
60. Reitan K. The initial tissue reaction incident to orthodontic tooth movement as related to the influence of function: an experimental histologic study on animal and human material. Acta Odontol Scand Suppl. 1951;6:1–240.
61. Reitan K, et al. Tissue rearrangement during retention of orthodontically rotated teeth. Angle Orthod. 1959;29:105–13.
62. Reitan K. Principles of retention and avoidance of posttreatment relapse. Am J Orthod. 1969;55:776–90.
63. Little RM, et al. Serial extraction of first premolars-postretention evaluation of stability and relapse. Angle Orthod. 1990;60:255–62.
64. Brodie AG. Consideration of musculature in diagnosis, treatment, and retention. Am J Orthod. 1952;38:823–35.
65. Proffit WR. Equilibrium theory revisited: factors influencing position of the teeth. Angle Orthod. 1978;48:175–86.
66. Strang RHW. The fallacy of denture expansion as a treatment procedure. Angle Orthod. 1949;19:12–22.

67. King GJ, et al. Alveolar bone turnover and tooth movement in male rats after removal of orthodontic appliances. Am J Orthod Dentofac Orthop. 1997;111:266–75.
68. McManus A, et al. Evaluation of BSP expression and apoptosis in the periodontal ligament during orthodontic relapse: a preliminary study. Orthod Craniofac Res. 2014;17(4):239–48.
69. Franzen TJ, et al. Expression of bone markers and micro-CT analysis of alveolar bone during orthodontic relapse. Orthod Craniofac Res. 2014;17(4):249–58.
70. Yadav S, et al. The effect of low-frequency mechanical vibration on retention in an orthodontic relapse model. Eur J Orthod. 2015;38(1):44–50.

Tooth Movement Mechanobiology: Toward a Unifying Concept

2

Donald J. Ferguson and M. Thomas Wilcko

Abstract

Tooth movement, as it is generally visualized by orthodontist clinicians, is modeled as a biological event mediated by the cells of the periodontal ligament (PDL) whereby alveolar bone resorption is witnessed on the "pressure" side and bone apposition on the "tension" side. This "pressure-tension" image is burned so deeply into the orthodontic psyche after a century plus of scrutiny that the structural features, characteristics, and mechanisms involving the tooth, the PDL, and the alveolar bone are at the heart of the prevailing tooth movement paradigm and have dominated investigatory attention. Scholarship on tooth movement biology has focused on breaking down the cell-centric "pressure-tension" model into its component parts so as to tease out individual functions. Our understanding of the tissue, cellular, and molecular mechanisms involved in orthodontic tooth movement has created a segregated literature and knowledge base of part-processes that is indeed impressive. But these reductionist explanations of the physical body – this collection of parsed physiological processes – have not resulted in a cohesive understanding of clinically relevant tooth movement.

During the past 15 years, interest in accelerating tooth movement has grown. The common basis for biologically based acceleration techniques is some form of injury to the alveolus resulting in mineralized tissues surrounding the teeth becoming less mineralized (osteopenia). It is the increase in tissue turnover and the osteopenia of alveolar trabecular bone that facilitates rapid tooth movement. Lessons learned from acceleration technique wound healing draws attention to

D.J. Ferguson, DMD, MSD (✉)
Department of Orthodontics, European University College, Dubai Healthcare City, Dubai, United Arab Emirates
e-mail: fergusonloud@gmail.com

M.T. Wilcko, DMD
Private Practice in Periodontology, Erie, PA, USA

Department of Periodontology, Case Western Reserve University, Cleveland, OH, USA

B. Shroff (ed.), *Biology of Orthodontic Tooth Movement*,
DOI 10.1007/978-3-319-26609-1_2

the importance of tissue strain, microenvironments, and tissue turnover and brings us face-to-face with the body as lived in relationship to a changed environment. The intentionally injured body takes predictable actions through the sensing and interplay of multitudes of information for the sake of reestablishing equilibrium, and in this regard, the local-regional interpretation of microstrain means a lot. Mechanobiological disciplines like orthodontics are best understood through stresses imposed, strains experienced, and how the lived body – inseparable from its environment – intentionally adapts and reestablishes homeostasis.

Tooth movement biology, in order to be coherent, needs to be based upon an understanding of the mechanobiology that unfolds in the lived body actively engaged in immediate and meaningful interaction with the environment with the intended goal of achieving/maintaining homeostasis. In the humble opinion of the authors, a shift toward an understanding of intentional relations in nature, i.e., the mechanical "thresholds" of microstrain that normal and repair tissues encounter for different in vivo activities, is critically important in understanding tooth movement and moves us toward a unifying "phenomenological" concept of tooth movement biology. Tooth movement is unique; what emerges as critical in an understanding of these phenomena is the extraordinary sensitivity of trabecular bone anabolic and catabolic modeling to a combination of strain and the influence of intramedullary pressure changes on bone fluid flow. The present day inability to measure strain and pressure accurately in the various microenvironments involved in tooth movement is a hiccup worth overcoming.

2.1 Prevailing TM Paradigm: An Account

2.1.1 Current Paradigm

Tooth movement as currently understood from a "wet-fingered" clinical perspective is that when an orthodontic appliance applies a force, there is little movement initially but after a month or so teeth begin to move. A clinician's understanding is that of a cell-mediated process – that the periodontal ligament (PDL) experiences "pressure" in the direction of movement and "tension" on the opposite side. The PDL is recognized as the major site of activity with some contribution from undermining resorption on the medullary side of the lamina dura [88, 105]. This model is uncomplicated and visual, explains and predicts tooth movement based upon over a century of observations, aids in clinical decision making, and can be comprehended in its entirety because this pressure-tension model contains only those structure and process features that are of primary importance. Teeth move at a rate that is somewhat predictable, comprehensive orthodontic treatment takes 21–27 months for non-extraction therapy and 25–35 months for extraction treatment [10].

Less familiar to the nonacademic orthodontic clinician but nevertheless accepted and emerging is the mechanobiological model of tooth movement in which strain (deformation) is perceived and adaptive mechanisms affecting mineralized and non-mineralized paradental tissues eventually bring the host back to steady-state homeostasis [24, 54]. Teeth move orthodontically through the alveolar bone because mechanical stress (load) results in strain (deformation) within a cell-rich viscoelastic system. Strain in hydrodynamic closed or semi-closed biological systems leads to cellular responses with feedback controls, and these physiological regulatory processes stabilize health and functioning [47]. Sustained stresses to the dentoalveolar complex can come from orthodontic force application (intentional) or injury (intentional or unintentional) and both are examples of external stimuli (stresses) resulting in biological strain and the initiation of physiological regulatory processes that eventually return tissues to an active and sensitive steady-state condition.

2.1.2 Evolution of Tooth Movement Concept: A Typological Account

The prevailing PDL cell-mediated pressure-tension paradigm is firmly rooted in the structure and process features of tooth movement. Hence, an evolutionary account of tooth movement concept based upon its features and characteristics, i.e., a typological account, appears relevant. The scholarly literature amassed to date describing tooth movement biology is impressive and diverse, and the literature base broadly coincides with the historical development of investigative techniques that have been applied to study tooth movement [21], i.e., light microscopy [96, 122], histomorphometry [109, 129], histochemistry [23], electron microscopy [118], in vitro culturing [68], and autoradiography [39], somewhat in that order; molecular biology has been dominate from the 1970s and computed tomography has developed since.

2.1.2.1 Histology to Histomorphometry

Comprehensive and detailed evolutionary accounts of tooth movement concepts are provided by others [21, 82, 102, 121]. The description provided here reviews the PDL cell-centric nature of these concepts that serve to predict how the microstructure and biological constitution of the tissues supporting tooth movement have evolved as a consequence of the mechanical environment.

The idea that orthodontic tooth movement is dependent on the cells responsible for resorption and deposition of the bone of the socket dates back at least to 1839 [82]. The prevailing cell-centric paradigm for the biology of tooth movement, however, was initialed in a three-part article on the theory of tooth movement published in 1904–1905 in which Sandstedt convincingly demonstrated, apparently for the first time, tooth movement as a process of resorption and apposition. Sandstedt described histologically and radiographically that "the (alveolar) wall appears to move" as apposition on the alveolar side is balanced by resorption in adjacent vascular spaces and vice versa. New bone formation was shown in areas of tension, and resorption was demonstrated in areas of compression (pressure zones); he provided a first description of a hyaline zone developed during tooth movement and notes that "at the limit of the hyaline zone the alveolar wall presents a deep, undermining notch filled by proliferating cells as in resorptive areas." His seminal work was followed in 1911 by Oppenheim with a description of tissue change incident to tooth movement particularly of the bone [82].

It was the histomorphometric descriptions in human tissues by Reitan that gained wide attention in 1950s and further elucidated an understanding of tooth movement highlighting tissue response based upon type and magnitude of force, type of tooth movement, and variability of tissue reactions between individuals. Storey added the concept of differential force application in the 1950s and the idea that there is an optimum range of force values that will produce the maximum rate of tooth movement. Autoradiography was introduced in the 1960–1970s to measure changes in cell proliferation and metabolic activity [21].

When mechanically loaded, it was described in the 1960s that the periodontal tissues behave as a viscoelastic gel which flows when subjected to a steady force but "bounces" when a load is briefly applied and then removed [82]. In the 1960s and 1970s, attention was drawn to the effects of bone bending on tooth movement and the physiological strain magnitude on changes in metabolic activity with later interest in the molecular. The in vitro cell and tissue culture systems of the 1970s provided some answers to questions not readily accessible from animal studies conducted in vivo [82]. Davidovitch [21] reviewed the evolution of concepts regarding the biological foundation of force-induced tooth movement and described the known mechanobiological regulation involved at that period of time.

2.1.2.2 Molecular Mechanisms

During the 1970s, the mechanobiological pressure-tension model was well established as it became more apparent that mechanical strain activates multiple cell internal signaling pathways and/or second messengers in order to modulate the behavior of all cells responsible for tooth movement within the hydrodynamic periodontal ligament and alveolar bone [82]. Knowledge of these molecular signaling systems in the biomedical sciences exploded at an alarming rate during the "long 1970s [130]."

Krishnan [61, 62] expanded the overview of the orthodontic tooth movement process, by delineating reactions occurring in mineralized (alveolar bone) and non-mineralized (PDL and gingiva) paradental tissues and their associated neurovascular networks. The authors presented known information about the mechanism of cell signaling in response to mechanical loading, including mechanosensing, transduction, and cellular responses. They presented the various components of this extracellular matrix (ECM)/cellular interrelated chain of responses in an organized sequence, highlighting the links between clinical events and knowledge derived from basic research [62].

2.1.2.3 Mechanobiology

Mechanobiology is the understanding of biology from the perspective of mechanics and how physical forces influence the movement of molecules in cells, the molecular mechanisms by which cells sense and respond to mechanical signals (mechanotransduction), how cells know when and how much to differentiate, and to where cells migrate [25]. For the musculoskeletal system, mechanobiology is the understanding of how skeletal tissues are produced, maintained, and adapted as an active response to biophysical stimuli in their environment [24].

Cell-centric mechanobiological models, i.e., the view that cell-level effects will be extrapolated directly to the tissue or organ, have been used to describe tooth movement after orthodontic force application [21, 53, 61, 62, 77, 78, 81, 82, 139, 152, 155]. But the cell-centric model of tooth movement that has been our history does not fully account for clinical observations.

There is an incomplete understanding of bone and PDL tissue adaptation (turnover) but skeletal turnover encompasses modeling and remodeling, a complex network of cell–cell and cell–matrix interactions involving systemic hormones, locally produced cytokines, and growth factors, many of which are sequestrated within the bone matrix, as well as the mechanical environment of the cells [82, 121]. Calcified bone matrix of the lamina dura and trabecular bone must become decalcified by osteoclasts in order for a tooth to change in position [144], and it is well known but poorly understood how osteocytes initiate and control bone turnover [53, 54] and how the development and activity of osteoclasts are under the control of the osteoblasts [45].

Biophysical and biochemical tooth movement mechanisms have been intensely studied, yet the links between tissue response and force application remain obscure. It is fair to say that reductionist strategies have been used in an effort to understand the complex phenomenon called tooth movement [82], i.e., by analyzing what is considered the basic mechanisms or the essences of the topic [17]. Our ability to identify, catalogue, and classify events that affect the sequence, timing, and significance of factors that determine the nature of the biological response of each paradental tissue to orthodontic force is quite impressive [62]. But so doing in this manner identifies us as typological and does not take into account the particular kinds of variation exhibited by individuals that are a concrete feature of the world that has primacy in biological theorizing [72].

The pressure-tension concept is currently, and has been, the essence of and central to explanations of tooth movement [105, 139]. Meikle [82] indicated that the idea that pressure and tension sites are generated within the PDL is firmly embedded in the orthodontic subconscious and it continues to play a key role in organizing our ideas, as well as advancing our understanding of a complex biological process. After 100+ years, the orthodontic community has a reasonably good understanding of the sequence of events involved in orthodontic tooth movement at the tissue and cellular levels on both the tensile and compression sides of the periodontium [82]. Scholarly literature suggests that much is known about bone apposition and resorption and "that" understanding explains tooth movement.

But have we not been answering an easier question than the one that needs to be answered [120]? In our search for a means to fulfill our need to understand, we end up answering not "What explains tooth movement?" but rather the more tractable "What inherent features of the pressure-tension event explains tooth movement"? The latter question focuses on what we already know, i.e., inherence heuristic and cognitive processes that appeal to the inherent features [120] of the pressure-tension concept; the former question does not. There is no rational basis for preferring an explanation of tooth movement based upon the properties of PDL pressure-tension. Is it not an obvious fact of perception that, if there is a change in the perspective of an object being viewed, the appearance of the object will change accordingly? [117] It is suggested that a more cogent explanation for tooth movement resides not from parsed processes of the physical body, but rather in a deeper understanding of biological stress and strain, i.e., the lived body in relation to its environment [151].

2.1.2.4 Tooth Movement Model Critique

According to Weiss et al. [150], inductive reasoning and hypothesis-driven experimentation are the driving forces behind reductionism ("bottom-up" research) in medical science. Reductionist scientists break down the proposed system into its component parts so as to tease out individual functions. Using this method, the system is viewed as equaling the sum of the parts and understanding the system as a whole depends on defining the important interactions of each of the system's constituents. A reductionist's approach to bone pathophysiology would entail, for example, breaking bone down into its component parts—the osteoblast, osteocyte, and osteoclast—and then determining the individual cell's function and the interactions it has with its neighbors. This would yield information that can be applied to produce a larger system of bone remodeling [150]. But an organism cannot be understood as a collection of individual parts, a concept contrary to reductionism, i.e., the entire patient (and not just the region of interest) and their milieu must be considered [151] because the stress–strain of biological tissues must be considered collectively. In other words, nature consists in relationships – it is a dynamic system of interdependencies not a collection of separate things [46], i.e., stress results in strain and strain results in a continuum of adaptive changes while the lived body seeks homeostasis.

Meikle [82] described as "reductionist" the chronological accounts of tooth movement focused on discovery of new molecules and experimental techniques and pointed out that doing so made the subject less accessible to the clinician. A review of orthodontic literature through the 2000s [47, 62, 63, 77, 78, 82, 139, 156] is testimony to the fact that reductionist explanations of tooth movement focused on molecular systems have not resulted in a cohesive understanding of clinically relevant tooth movement. The literature complied related to tissue, cellular, and molecular mechanisms involved in orthodontic tooth movement is extensive, but a coherent narrative on tooth movement biology does not exist [82]. In order for basic, mechanistic knowledge derived from "bottom-up" research to be effectively translated, the reductionist-derived knowledge must be placed back into a clinical context [145] and the way to do so is to decode the stress–strain dynamics of living tissues and consider the human body as inseparable from its environment.

The pressure-tension model, as represented in the scholarly literature, is depicted as a natural physical event. Orthodontists heretofore regard pressure-tension as an event that is characterized by osteoclastic resorption on the pressure side and osteoblastic apposition on the tension side – that to understand these essentials is to understand tooth movement [105]. Such a view of the pressure-tension construct is spatiotemporally restricted to the PDL and is insensitive to tissue strain variation except that too much biomechanical force will hyalinize the PDL and inhibit tooth movement for a time.

Biology examines the physical body, whereas phenomenology examines the body as a vehicle of lived experience [151]. Organisms live and operate as wholes and cannot be reduced to its smallest divisible units without losing something essential and meaningful from the whole; moreover, nothing can remain unchanged by a change in its environment [151]. In the context of the present discussion, it has been our history to model tooth movement activities based upon samples of physical data of the objective body using the cell-mediate PDL pressure-tension model. The method of reducing an organism to its smallest parts suggests that part-processes behave the same way regardless of context – a position which fails to understand meaningful deviations in such behavior [151]. To date, tooth movement scholarship has evolved primarily from third-person research methods of the physical or natural body and not from first-person investigation techniques of the body as lived. A first-person view of tooth movement may yield outcomes that do not behave the way mechanical phenomena do [117].

2.1.3 Beyond the Current Model

Cells convert mechanical signals into a biochemical response, but little is known about how they function in the structural context of living cells, tissues, and organs to produce orchestrated changes in cell behavior in response to stress. Ingber [56] suggested that our bodies use structural hierarchies (systems within systems) composed of interconnected extracellular matrix and cytoskeletal networks that span from the macroscale to the nanoscale to focus stresses on specific mechanotransducer molecules. A key feature of these networks is that they are in a state of isometric tension, i.e., experience a tensile prestress, which ensures that various molecular-scale mechanochemical transduction mechanisms proceed simultaneously and produce a concerted response. These features of living architecture are the same principles that govern tensegrity (tensional integrity) architecture, and mathematical models based on tensegrity are beginning to provide new and useful descriptions of living materials, including mammalian cells [56].

The body is a physical thing, an object that can be weighed, measured, and described using purely physical or naturalistic terms. But the body is also a perceiving and experiencing organism actively engaged in immediate and meaningful interaction with the environment in order to achieve/maintain homeostasis, i.e., the lived body [151]. The body as lived, or the habitual body, is a relationship to an environment and to a set of abilities [11]. Actions take place constantly through the sensing and interplay of multitudes of information for the sake of maintaining/achieving equilibrium. These interactions with the environment are inhabited by meaning; the body executes goal-directed actions that reflect the visible form of its global and meaningful intentions [11]. This embodied phenomenology or phenomenal body is a unified potential or capacity to achieve/maintain homeostasis.

There are unique features about the physical environment where tooth movement takes place. The fibrous joint between tooth and bone is specialized and persists life-long. The periodontal ligament (PDL) that provides support, sensory, nutritive, and renewal functions is biologically unique. The PDL width ranges from 0.15 to 0.38 mm and consists of 53–74 % collagen fibers and 1–2 % blood vessels and nerve endings embedded into an amorphous mucopolysaccharide matrix [99]. The PDL is about 70 % water in a viscoelastic system which helps teeth to withstand stress loads [93, 94, 128]. Fibroblasts are the principle cell of the PDL and occupy about 20–35 % of the ligament volume, excluding the blood vessels [147]. PDL fibroblasts are highly sensitive to mechanical stress and are responsible for the rapid turnover of their extracellular compartment, collagen, which allows a rapid adaptation of the tissue to changing loads, such as in orthodontic tooth movement [147]. Collagen fiber bundles end in either the cementum or embedded in the bundle bone of the lamina dura, i.e., Sharpey's fibers [93, 94]. The PDL may be loaded under a long-lasting, sustained force system (orthodontics) or under short-term, impact-type force applications (mastication). Viscoelastic properties are dependent on the magnitude and the frequency of the loads applied [99].

Alveolar bone is comprised of cortical bone with compact structures and low porosity that forms the hard shell and trabecular bone with a three-dimensional interconnected network of trabecular rods and plates that forms the inner surface. The cortical bone haversian system with osteocytes and complex, diverse types of branching, and interconnections consists of repeating osteons averaging in diameter about 200 μm. In trabecular bone, the trabecular rods and plates form three-dimensional structures, and within the trabeculae are less regular arranged lamellae and osteocytes. The main components of bone matrix are organic material (10–30 % in amount) and mineral salts (70–90 % in amount). The organic material, which is primarily type I collagen (90 %) and nonfibrillar organic matrix (osteocalcin and osteopontin present in a large proportion) gives the bone toughness. The mineral salts, mainly nanocrystallite apatite materials, permeate the organic matrix and provide the characteristic rigidity and strength of bone [110]. The trabecular bone is subject to strain while surrounded by marrow that is a highly viscous fluid; experimental studies have shown that loading of bone induces pressure gradients within the marrow, known as the intramedullary pressure [6, 86]. Hence, the medullary space is an interesting mechanobiological microenvironment comprised of trabecular bone displaying poroelastic properties and subject to strain as well as bone marrow displaying properties of a viscoelastic solid and subject to intramedullary pressure changes [6].

In structural connective tissues, loads are carried not by the cells themselves but by the extracellular matrix (ECM) which they produce [49, 57]. ECM components, which fill the space around cells in the periodontal ligament, are mainly composed of fibrous molecules and ground substance. The major fibrous molecules are type I and type III collagens which play a main role in resisting tensional forces and holding teeth in the alveolar socket [98]. For collagen from fibroblasts, various types and orientations are produced [94], and for bone from osteoblasts, osteoid, woven, and lamellar bone provide varying degrees of structure and mineralization; the anisotropic properties of collagen and bone increase tissue strength. The tissues' ability to sustain functional loading without failure or damage is therefore achieved because the fibroblast matrix producing cells can regulate the orientation, mass, and physical properties (strength and stiffness) of their matrix in relation to the requirements of prevailing functional load-bearing [118]. Mechanical force is directly exerted on the periodontal ligament during orthodontic treatment, and periodontal ligament cells undergo great changes in morphology and function, leading to active degradation and synthesis of extracellular matrix [13, 98]. Stiffness of the PDL increases with increasing loading velocity [13, 98].

The periodontal ligament plays important roles in mediation of mechanical force, in alveolar bone modeling and remodeling and in maintenance of physiologic equilibrium within periodontal tissue [13]. PDL collagens type I and type III produced from fibroblasts are the major fibrous molecules that play an important role in resisting tensional forces [58], and in the homeostatic PDL, the ratio of type I to type III is approximately 5 to 1 [137]. The collagen-type balance changes in acute phases of inflammation and healing with type III collagen synthesized in excess of type I collagen, while type I synthesis predominates in the fibrosis stage of inflammation [137].

Compositions of the various microenvironments are altered as a consequence of sustained (especially episodic) stress, i.e., more type III collagen in strained PDL [13] or higher percentage of woven compared to lamella bone in the medullary space [13]. Fibroblast-sourced progenitor cells in the periodontal ligament can differentiate into osteoblasts for the physiological maintenance of alveolar bone [49, 58, 111, 147]. Collagen fiber bundles are basic guarantees for osteoblast phenotype and calcium nodule formation and their characteristics, to a certain extent, determine bone formation. If fiber bundles are bulky and dense, bony tissue will deposit along the stretched fiber bundles and be embedded in the fiber bundles to form the lamellar bone. If fiber bundles are thin, bony tissue will evenly deposit on the bone surface [13].

PDL mechanics cannot be expected to be as simple as a crystalline material such as bone [94]. Soft tissues such as the PDL exhibit complex constitutive behavior, being viscoelastic, inhomogeneous, anisotropic, and nonlinear, and exhibit a susceptibility to irreversible damage during the initial cycles of loading [94], i.e., "preconditioning" or "strain softening." The PDL in vivo will stiffen under conditions of sustained stress [99] in order to reduce future strain levels and the elastic modulus will vary with strain rate with steeper stress–strain curve at higher strain rate. PDL modulus of elasticity is so low compared to elastic modulus of teeth and cortical bone that an order of magnitude variance in the PDL modulus of elasticity from 6 to 12 MPa due to PDL composition change does not make much of a difference on these tissues with a modulus about 35 times greater [116]. However alveolar trabecular bone beyond the lamina dura has a modulus similar to the PDL and is quite sensitive to changes in stress; strains of 0.2 % or 2000 microstrain initiates turnover changes in trabecular bone [90].

2.1.3.1 Bone Modeling and Remodeling

Bones of the skeleton are designed to provide structure, and tissue strain is likely the most relevant parameter to control. And vice versa, strain, or its immediate consequence, is the load-related event most likely to influence bone cell behavior and therefore bone structure. Strain distribution is a controlling variable for functional adaptation in bone tissue and adaptive bone change will be stimulated by strain situations where the strains are not abnormally high, but simply "inappropriately" distributed. Mechanically adaptive bone modeling is sensitive to both strain distribution and strain magnitude. An increase in strain level, if sustained, will result in an increase in bone mass and/or structural rearrangement, and hence an increase in bone strength [118, 135].

Bone experiences internal strain when mechanically loaded (stressed), and from an engineering standpoint, strain refers to the change in length of a bone (deformation) when load is applied. As mentioned previously, strain is a unit-less value, and strain is small for bone and often expressed in terms of microstrain or $\mu\varepsilon$ [34, 148]. Strains in living bone result in bone formation and/or resorption, and these basic metabolic processes are cell-level activities conducted by osteoblasts and osteoclasts. However, the type and function of the bone at the tissue level, whether it be cortical bone or trabecular bone, will dictate transduction signaling mechanisms, feedback loops, and physiological processes within microenvironments at all organizational levels from nano-level to organ-level. How bone metabolizes depends upon strain level and homeostatic demands of that particular cortical or trabecular bone microenvironment, i.e., bone remodeling and modeling [24, 30, 113, 114].

There are important differences between bone modeling and bone remodeling, and these differences, although controversial, are seldom discerned in discussions about tooth movement. Bone modeling is a bone surface activity that leads to shape, mass, and strength changes [4, 28, 34, 108, 110, 126]. Where dynamic strain threshold exceeds the skeletal tissue's minimum effective strain for modeling, i.e., >1000–1500 microstrain ($\mu\varepsilon$), mechanically controlled surface changes of cortical and trabecular bone is turned on (lamellar or layered bone apposition); modeling involves adding more tissue or changing the structure's micro- and macro-architecture and/or shape, thereby increasing local-regional bone strength and stiffness with the net effect of reducing tissue strain [30]. Both anabolic and catabolic bone modeling results from a stimulus representing activation, and the mechanisms are independent processes (uncoupled) from each other [16, 53, 59].

In contrast, bone remodeling is a bone subsurface activity that leads to renewal of haversian bone and, in healthy adults, results in a zero-based exchange, i.e., causes neither gains nor losses of bone. Where dynamic strains exceed the skeletal tissue's minimal effective strain for remodeling threshold (<100 $\mu\varepsilon$), remodeling is switched on and turns cortical bone over in small packets performed by specialized groups of cells (BMUs) comprised of cutting and filling cones, i.e., secondary osteon formation [59]. The sequence of events is coupled as activation < resorption < formation or A-R-F [24, 34, 59, 106], i.e., new bone is formed only on a previously resorbed surface. In the same macroscopic bone at the same time, modeling and remodeling can respond in opposite ways to the same stimulus, although both mechanisms appear to utilize the same kinds of osteoblasts and osteoclasts [37].

The tooth movement that is achieved after sustained force application is a consequence of strain perceived and a complex orchestration of events that appear to be dependent upon the rate-limiting temporal dynamics of the periodontal ligament (PDL) and its contents, i.e., immediate PDL compression <4-week lag time for a local PDL bone modeling cell population shift and mobilization sufficient to induce tooth movement<indefinite frontal resorption as well as undermining resorption with tooth movement of 1 mm per month (for translation type movement). However, according to Frost, the basis for understanding this phenomenon does not equate to mechanical stress acting upon effector cells leading to tooth movement, but rather on an understanding of how strain acts at other organizational levels which he termed the intermediary organization [30]. The lamina dura immediately adjacent to the PDL is cortical bone and typical trabecular bone in the medullary cavity is not. Hence, there are two distinctive bone microenvironments involved in tooth movement leading to increased strain which respond differently, i.e., cortical bone (internal) remodeling does not increase significantly, while trabecular bone (surface) modeling activity increases dramatically.

The prevailing pressure-tension event model is typological and flawed. Orthodontic research is misguided when using pressure-tension as a typological event [72]. Time and again the same statements are made in clinical study after clinical study as stated by Van Schepdael et al. [139], "Accurate prediction of orthodontic tooth movement is made difficult by the high inter-patient variability and by the complexity of the process." The classic, ongoing example of this is the optimal force question. It has been demonstrated in orthodontic literature that there are certain thresholds of orthodontic mechanical load application beyond which controlled tooth movement rate or magnitudes are not affected; the threshold in beagle dogs for moving second premolars into extraction sites was reported as 300 cN above which tooth movement rate was not affected [140]. While threshold levels reported have varied depending on the experimental animal used, the optimal force investigation has been pursued repeatedly and consistently decade after decade [2, 101, 107, 146] yielding the same results, i.e., beyond a certain threshold of force application, tooth movement rate is not affected. Substantial individual variation in treatment response is always observed and described (mentioned) in orthodontic force magnitude studies which cannot be explained by data gathered.

In general, a greater strain signal has a greater effect on bone formation and bone resorption, but for any given strain signal, the strain signal is lower in bones with greater mass and is higher in bones with less mass [6, 65]. Individual subject "robustness" represents variation in the strain response to the same level of stress and plays a significant role in explaining subject variation in controlled investigations such as optimal orthodontic force studies. In the opinion of the authors, a deeper understanding of the orchestrating nature of tissue strain within the two unique bone microenvironments in tooth movement (cortical versus trabecular) should explain the inter-patient variability cited. Application of orthodontic forces generates bone strain levels and hydrostatic pressures greater than "steady state" and initiates an adaptive response from bone; that response is in the form of primarily catabolic and anabolic modeling with the purpose of increasing strength and/or physiological competence and reducing strain back toward "steady-state" levels [37].

A strain-centric model for tooth movement would include controlled orthodontic mechanical load (stress) and tissue strain. The load increases deformation of both the extracellular matrix (substrate strain) and increases extracellular fluid flow [97]. Alveolar bone marrow is a highly vascularized with cellular soft tissues located in the medullary cavity and in the pore spaces of trabecular bone. Loading of whole bones leads to deformation which increases the interstitial bone fluid flow creating a hydraulic pressure gradient in the bone marrow, and marrow cells respond to these mechanical stimuli [106]. Stress in the trabecular bone marrow during loading reaches a sufficient magnitude to affect cell mechanobiology [86].

The initial localized mechanical signal to bone cells does not activate remodeling of cortical bone lamina dura, but the increased strain and hydrostatic pressure does activate both anabolic and catabolic uncoupled lamina dura and trabecular modeling. The initial applied orthodontic force induces a decrease in strain (<100 με) on the side of tooth movement and lamina dura remodeling is activated [83]; at the same time, extracellular tissue flow increases microstrain within the medullary cavity on the side toward the tooth movement. Catabolic modeling takes place on the medullary surface of the lamina dura on the side of tooth movement in response to reduced strain and resulting in undermining resorption; uncoupled anabolic modeling within the medullary cavity on the side of movement responds to increased medullary cavity hydraulic pressure (>3000 με) resulting in woven bone production, medullary stiffening, and an increase in overall or whole-bone strength and toughness. By the time the lamina dura has demineralized on the side of movement by a combination of remodeling and catabolic modeling, trabecular bone has transitioned from lamellar to predominately woven bone which has unique material and mechanical characteristics (dense, tough and resists resorption). The former strength provided by the lamina dura has been replaced with a medullary cavity dominated by woven bone formation on the side of movement [83] inspired by an increased hydraulic pressure gradient [106] and medullary pressure from extracellular fluid flow and whole-bone competence.

2.1.3.2 A Phenomenological TM Concept

An organism's biology is best understood when it is recognized that the organism and environment mutually participate in the event of actualization [151]. Hanley [46] described intentional relations in nature as phenomenology applied to the natural sciences and Goldstein used the equation [phenomenon = organism + environment] to explain interventions [151]. A mechanobiological approach describes the evolution of the structure and biological constitution, whereas a phenomenological approach describes the global mechanical behavior [85]. A phenomenological orthodontic equation should be tooth movement = load applied + tissue strain. In tooth movement, stress (load) and strain (deformation) are intentional, simultaneous, and reciprocally related. The organism changes and the environment changes and vice versa; both must be consulted for understanding the biological event [151]. The declaration that "the stress-generated signals that are so important for normal function have little if anything to do with the response to tooth movement" [105] is misinformed and ill-advised; orthodontically generated stress signals represent a deviation from the typical prestress of daily living.

In orthodontic tooth movement, the environment within which the tooth movement takes place is meaningful to that activity – it is an example of the lived body relating to its environment [46] and best described by stress and strain as the essential characteristics. A collection of pressure-tension descriptions is not the essence of understanding tooth movement – tissue strain and the lived body strength needed to adapt to the orthodontic load is. This "tissue strain" notion of pressure-tension invites, no… requires a consideration of strain variation within microenvironments because the events that unfold using stress–strain dynamics must be in the context of how much stress is employed, how much strain experienced per microenvironment, and the ever-changing temporal strength adaptations taking place. The principal context is a lived body striving to reach equilibrium (homeostasis); it seems fruitless to try and build a compelling tooth movement model short of the inseparable combination of orthodontic load + tissue strain relative to the unique microenvironments involved.

We believe a rational understanding of "optimal" tooth movement resides in the ever-changing dynamic relationship of microstrain in the microenvironments involved, and it is only when these relationships are deciphered will a unifying concept of tooth movement emerge. Mechanical loads are applied at the organ-level and propagate to a level where cells can sense them; forces define much of the organization of cells [29] which in turn results in changes at the tissue level [5]. The lived body and its networks are in a constant state of isometric tension or tensile prestress (tensional integrity) in response to daily activities, gravity, etc. [56]. Mechanical stress (load) from an orthodontic appliance creates tissue-/cell-level strain beyond typical daily living leading to an increase in hard and soft tissue turnover. Strain is a unit-less value often expressed in terms of microstrain or με wherein 0.1 % deformation = 1000 με. The various tissues involved in tooth movement are more or less sensitive to strain changes, for example, contents of the PDL turnover at low, i.e., ~1500 με [116], trabecular bone responds to all levels of microstrain [15, 90], and cortical bone remodels at very low microstrain levels, i.e., <50 με [34, 142], <100 με [59] or <100–300 με [83].

The tooth movement itself perpetuates strain until the tooth stops moving and malocclusion is resolved, and the host continues to adapt during the process. Hence, tooth movement from sustained tissue strain within the periodontium is unique and represents a complicated "quantum" process of energy dissipation requiring changes in the PDL as well as the supporting alveolar bone, tissues with different cell populations, and modeling/remodeling (turnover) characteristics.

In the dog study [140], it would appear that the orthodontic loads of 300 and 500 cN were interpreted by the host tissues with a certain degree of sameness and that "sameness" may have been due to woven bone modeling. In all likelihood, local remodeling effector cells were turned off while modeling effector cells for woven bone were turned on, especially at the 300–500 cN load range. Woven bone is produced when microstrain levels are >3000 με [43] and/or when bone strength needs to increase immediately, but this partially mineralized tissue is somewhat resorption resistant and it takes time for lamellar bone replacement. Moreover, hydraulic stiffening of marrow within the trabecular bone compartments of whole bones provides additional stiffness to the overall bone [6]. In the orthodontic mechanical load studies cited, there was no accounting for whole-bone strength or robustness. The host responds to stress through a series of adaptive responses that help thwart future stress and, for skeletal tissue, that means anabolic modeling to increase bone strength [59]. If 300 and 500 cN loads elicit similar host responses, tooth movement rate is not affected. In this context, human physiology uses early environmental cues in preparing responses to future life experiences [133] and homeostasis is brought into the conversation. This is a phenomenological explanation based upon host stress plus tissue strain and does not encompass any particular underlying mechanism in physical, chemical, or molecular terms [5]. And this explanation also raises issues with regards to spatial and temporal scaling and dynamic changes within unique microenvironments as there are no governing principles that serve to explain except for a strain-centric model.

2.2 Lessons Learned from Wound Healing

Intentionally wounding, such is in surgical intervention, changes the equilibrium of local tissue fluids and results in transient swelling and edema. Bone tissue contains two types of fluid, blood, and interstitial fluid. Interstitial flow is considered to have a role in bone's mechanosensory system [19, 67]. Interstitial fluid flow in bone results from transcortical (intramedullary) pressure gradients produced by vascular and hydrostatic pressure [52]; both hydrostatic pressure and mechanical loading serve to mediate injury-induced anabolic and catabolic bone changes [22, 48]. When tissue injury occurs, the equilibrium balance between intra- and extracellular fluid compartments can no longer be sustained, and the increases in the pressure or velocity of bone fluid flow act to enhance mechanotransductory signaling and anabolic bone modeling [51]. This has been demonstrated using dynamic hydraulic stimulation, i.e., increased compression from a cuff placed over a limb, which resulted in increased bone fluid flow and increased anabolic trabecular bone modeling within 24–48 h of compression application [50].

Experimental orthodontics resulting in accelerated tooth movement has raised awareness that the prevailing PDL cell-centric paradigm of tooth movement does not satisfactorily explain the biological changes observed when the periodontium is stimulated by a noxious insult like corticotomy. PDL cell mediation and undermining resorption do not readily explain observations following intentional alveolar injury. Explanations are inadequate for observations such as translation of a canine into a first premolar extraction site at the rate of 6 mm per month (dental distraction), or active orthodontic treatment times averaging 6 months (selective alveolar decortication). Attempting to explain what happens to the cell-mediated PDL tooth movement model when the alveolus is intentionally wounded offers important insight into the biology of tooth movement. Only when a model cannot adequately explain the experimental data set or observations, a refinement of the model together with a change in model parameters seems appropriate [141].

2.2.1 A Focus on Wound Healing

Wounding, and the tissue strains and intramedullary pressures that ensue, forces an understanding of the interplay between space and time. Wound healing is a clear example of spatial processing and represents a continuum or gradient from acute tissue turnover to steady-state homeostasis depending upon the magnitude of the wound and the distance from the site of injury; the uniqueness of the physiological activity along that physical continuum is time-bound beginning from injury occurrence [87]. Biological systems and the cells that compose them have finite size and age features, and decisions such as "when" to stop growing and "when" to divide are also inherently "where" questions [26]. A stem cell, for example, has no need to differentiate and divide if it is sitting within an intact tissue, but as the needs of the tissue change or as nearby damaged tissues are encountered, new growth becomes necessary; continuously monitoring the spatial environment ensures that the mechanisms inherent to cellular processes can be timed appropriately [26]. From the cell's perspective, the local pressures and strain field and how it changes from the baseline condition is what drives adaptation; it is unlikely that the direction of loading is important [79]. Hence, a fuller understanding of tooth movement should emerge if there is a shift in focus from a cell-centric to strain-centric concept.

2.2.1.1 Strain

The magnitude of bone forming and resorbing events are controlled by intramedullary pressure or pressure gradients in the marrow milieu as it has been demonstrated that controlled enhancement of intramedullary pressure results in significantly increased trabecular bone anabolic and catabolic modeling [149]. Although a positive effect of hydrostatic pressure on bone formation has been identified [50], the exact value of that pressure in human bone tissue has not been determined in vivo. The strains are amplified locally and the local strain maxima will constitute the true effective strain [110].

Wounding causes tissue strain and there is widespread evidence, both clinical and laboratory-based, that bone healing depends on the mechanical conditions at the injury site [87]. Tissue strain is generated because of a combination of inflammatory processes and the closed or semi-closed hydrodynamic nature of host tissues [24, 110]. Level of mechanical injury stress applied at the time at wounding can be measured experimentally, but quantifying tissue strain and hydrostatic pressure is more complex and study of healing tissues characteristics have depended, for the most part, on information derived using finite element modeling [110, 141]. Although strain levels within tissues after wounding is not easily quantified [86, 87, 146], response to the tissue strain incurred from injury has been analyzed using high-resolution peripheral quantitative computed tomography technology, i.e., assessment of in vivo bone density, and architectural and mechanical properties at the microscale level [22].

When wounding bone introduces tissue strain levels exceeding >3000 $\mu\varepsilon$, there is an instant reduction in bone strength, and the time course of the change in bone strength and other biomechanical parameters has been calculated in humans by micro-finite element analysis [22]. Using the strain-centric concept, host response after wounding bone is focused on increasing bone strength in order to reduce healing strain levels, assure structural integrity and physiological competence, and eventually achieve maintenance strain levels consistent with homeostasis [118]. At tissue strain levels >3000 με, cortical bone remodeling does not contribute to increased bone strength and increased cortical anabolic modeling adds little bone strength [34]. However, increased intramedullary pressure gradients result in a rapid and extensive upregulation of trabecular anabolic modeling and serves as a primary source of increased bone strength and stiffness [22]. Trabecular bone is exquisitely sensitive to changes in mechanical environment, adaptive turnover is initiated at very small strain levels [15, 90], and woven bone production would be high following bone injury [22]. In a study of distal radius fracture healing in women, a 10 % decrease in bone stiffness was observed immediate post injury accompanied by about 10 % increase in trabecular thickness and density; the authors hypothesized that the formation of new woven bone in the trabecular region evident in the first weeks was the primary reason for the eventual post fracture improvement in bone strength [22]; woven bone mineralization is 50–70 % completed within a few days of apposition in humans and contributes significantly to bone stiffness, strength, and mechanical competence [4, 7, 20].

Lamellar bone is slowly formed in the adaptive threshold range (1000–2500 με), highly organized with parallel layers or lamellae that make it stronger (anisotropic property) than woven bone; woven bone is poorly organized with a more or less random arrangement of collagen fibers and mineral crystals [24, 138]. Woven bone forms as a dose-dependent response to tissue strain after wounding bone [73, 138, 155]. Woven bone is quickly formed when a threshold value of strain is exceeded [34, 134] and under conditions where a rapid rate of matrix deposition is needed [138]; the high strains associated with lamellar/woven bone transition has been estimated at ~5000 με [132]. Intramedullary woven bone forms de novo when mechanical strains were significantly elevated [9], a robust woven bone response can be expected within 7 days [73] after wounding and complete recovery of bone strength, and stiffness can be expected after 14 days [76] (Fig. 2.1).

2.2.1.2 Microenvironments

The ability to respond to injury and to repair is a fundamental property of almost all tissues, and two host characteristics during wound healing are important in an understanding of tissue strain reduction: microenvironments [87, 95, 121] and tissue turnover [29, 87], and both are best understood in the context of spatiotemporal scales [26]. The mechanical conditions local to the injury site, the strain microenvironments, are the stimuli responsible for guiding formation of different skeletal and nonskeletal tissues, and healing outcome is related to strain microenvironment; lower tensile strains are associated with bone formation [87]. The healing stages after wounding serve to refocus energy to reduce tissue strain by creating effective microenvironments that support essential functions [41, 44, 69, 75, 103, 126]. For example, aseptic inflammation and angiogenesis support increases in anabolic modeling which, in turn, increases bone strength and reduces local tissue strain. In self-limiting wound repair, host response varies according to distance from most severe

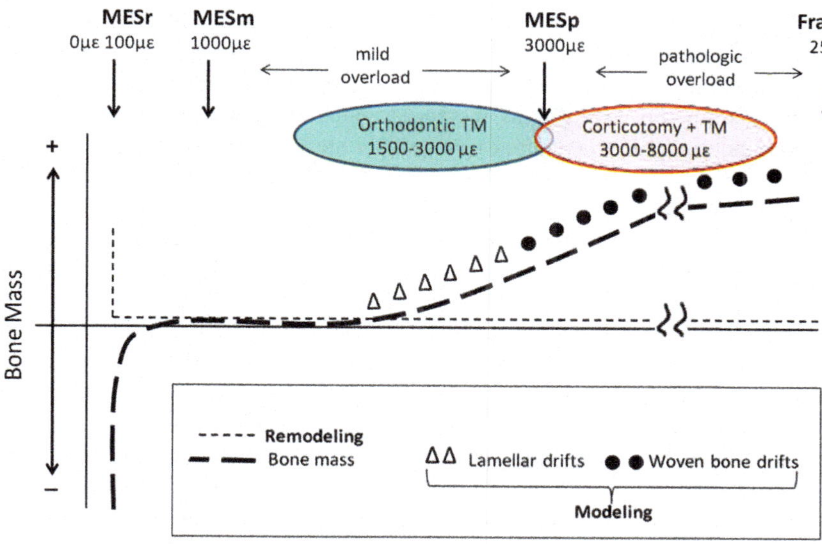

Fig. 2.1 A diagram illustrating the relationship of strains and adaptive responses. Note that osseous microstrain environment consistent with orthodontic tooth movement likely represented by 1500–3000 με and that alveolar corticotomy plus tooth movement is likely represented by 3000–8000 με (Redrawn and adapted from Jee [59])

injury scaled according to time since the injury occurred [29, 66, 125], and repair mechanisms and pathways are defined by the tissues of the microenvironment involved in the injury [95].

2.2.1.3 Turnover

Wound healing literature emphasizes the metabolic upregulation (turnover) of tissues, termed regional acceleratory phenomena or RAP, and microenvironments are affected along the spatiotemporal scale [29, 32, 33, 35, 142]. The catabolic and anabolic upregulation is very site-specific and only those regions within the individual loaded bone that experience sufficient microstrain adapt [34, 148]. Injury represents an abrupt external change forcing the host to seek a condition of equilibrium or stability within its internal environment (homeostasis) as a means of dealing with a noxa. Elevated strain in the range >1500 microstrain (με) results in increased activation frequency of modeling with more sites undergoing formation processes than resorption processes [8, 9]; lamellar apposition is less affected than woven bone formation when microstrain is >3000 με [80]. Histological evidence in long bone studies indicate that the cellular proliferation and angiogenic responses are different between conditions related to woven bone formation and conditions related to lamellar bone formation. The expression profiles demonstrate an earlier and more robust gene activation following higher tissue strains leading to woven bone formation and a later, lesser response following lower tissue strains leading to lamellar bone formation [80]. Hydrostatic pressure increases from intentional wounding, such as in the case of alveolar decortication, would result in dramatically increased anabolic modeling and woven bone production along a spatial gradient [83, 84] because cancellous bone is exquisitely sensitive to mechanical stimulation [15].

Elevated strain did not lead to increased remodeling activation resulting in increased bone mass nor was there evidence that elevated strain changes the individual vigor of osteoclasts or osteoblasts, or that the sigma period was altered [9]. As mentioned previously, in the same bone at the same time, modeling and remodeling can respond in opposite ways to the same stimulus [37]; microstrains >3000 $\mu\varepsilon$ turns on trabecular, periosteal, and endosteal modeling and turns off cortical haversian bone remodeling. There is a positive correlation between the initially applied peak strain and the rate of healing and bone stiffening [18].

Scales of space come into play because the intensity of the biological processes and physiological events (turnover) in host tissues decrease as a function of distance from the precise point or location of injury [29, 66, 125] and the spatial tissue gradient scale is influenced by the magnitude of the injury [87, 138]. The greatest tissue turnover (activity level) will be closest to the point of injury and the tissue turnover within that mechanical microenvironment is proportionate to injury magnitude [29, 155]. Formation of the different tissue types occurs in distinct strain microenvironments and the type of tissue formed is correlated most strongly to the local magnitudes of tissue strain [87]; that woven bone response that is scaled to the severity of injury indicates that woven bone formation is a well-regulated response to skeletal injury or to elevated mechanical strain [138].

2.2.2 Wound Healing and Orthodontic Tooth Movement in Perspective

Orthodontic force application resulting in tooth movement is a stimulus (arguably a mild form of wounding) that causes tissue strain at the >1000–2500 $\mu\varepsilon$ range, and repair processes are initiated purposefully aimed at returning the host to a state of homeostasis [128]. But tissue changes secondary to orthodontic mechanical stress are subtle compared to the scope and degree of tissue change subsequent to the stains introduced by tissue wounding of >3000 $\mu\varepsilon$. Wounding and orthodontic force application both create tissue strain, but the border between a noxa (wounding) and a mechanical stimulus (orthodontics) resulting in anabolic modeling has not yet been established [83]. The strain levels perceived as trauma are likely to be the same as the strain levels perceived as mechanical stress provoking a structural adaptation to mechanical usage [83]. The magnitude of tissue strain created by corticotomy surgery will exceed the tissue strain produced by orthodontic mechanical stress alone, i.e., the host response will be scaled to wounding strain levels and increased hydrostatic pressure, surgery site location, magnitude of surgical insult, and time; host response will not be scaled to orthodontic stress values.

In a wound, strain, and increased hydrostatic pressure are produced at the site of injury, bone healing depends on the mechanical conditions at the injury site [87]. At the cellular level, a wound forms a blood clot which initiates a cascade of events, including inflammation: immune cells arrive at the wound site to prevent infection and to remove debris followed by fibroblast proliferation, extracellular matrix (ECM) modeling, angiogenesis, and the deposition of new connective tissue, otherwise known as granulation tissue, a callus, or a scar [3, 104, 119, 127]. In healthy individuals who are injured, repair results in once functional tissue becoming a patch of cells, mainly fibroblasts, and disorganized extracellular matrix, mainly collagen [44]. In conventional orthodontic tooth movement, the mechanical stress is translated into tissue strain evoking an aseptic inflammatory response in the PDL microenvironment. And except for the clot formation, host response to orthodontic force application appears remarkably like the response to a wound leading to hyalinization followed by macrophage debris removal, angiogenesis, and revitalization of the PDL, but with a less intense spatiotemporal scale.

The microenvironments of particular interest in orthodontics are the PDL and trabecular bone which demand attention to principles of mechanobiology [74, 89]. If orthodontic tooth movement can be regarded as subclinical wounding, tooth movement secondary to reactivated orthodontic appliance adjustments has the effects of persistent wound signals invoking greater quantums of trabecular bone modeling activity [100] resulting in greater alveolar bone turnover [59, 142]. Verna and Melsen [144] manipulated alveolar bone turnover and reported greater rate and amount of tooth movement in high-turnover conditions [143, 144].

2.2.3 Alveolar Corticotomy and Orthodontics

Use of alveolar corticotomy to facilitate tooth movement dates back to late nineteenth century, but the treatment strategy lay fallow until the early 1950s when it was reintroduced as a corticotomy-osteotomy technique [60]. Alveolar corticotomy alone, i.e., without osteotomy, was reported in 1976 in the treatment of openbite malocclusion [40], and alveolar corticotomy with augmentation bone grafting was introduced in 2001 [92, 152, 153]. The effect of the combined hydrostatic pressure and tissue strain from selective alveolar decortication plus orthodontic force is unknown but strain most certainly exceeds the micro-damage range (>3000 $\mu\varepsilon$) compared to orthodontic treatment alone (1000–3000 $\mu\varepsilon$). Following alveolar decortication, catabolic modeling of trabecular bone and transient osteopenia in the medullary space [66, 125] serves to increase intramedullary pressure which further stimulates anabolic modeling and woven bone production [22]. Increased woven bone production [91] later remineralizes with no net bone matrix loss [66]; the time course for this is approximately 11 weeks in rats when no tooth movement is involved [125]. Trabecular bone is exquisitely sensitive to mechanical stimulation and suggests that the mechanical environment is a major determinant of the physiological behavior of mammalian cancellous bone [15]. Trabecular bone serves a metabolic function and turnover is very rapid following corticotomy [66, 112, 125]. Trabecular bone is also the tissue that, when calcified, serves as resistance or a barrier to tooth movement [143]. However, when the trabecular bone is demineralized, it is the closed or semi-closed hydrodynamic environment and the inherent strain-dependent signaling driven, in part, by moving teeth that controls rate and magnitude of tooth movement.

Given the complexity of the wound repair process, it is remarkable that repair rarely becomes uncontrolled [44, 64]. Wounded tissues change because there is continuing, persistent, declining strain and hydrostatic pressure until the system reaches steady-state equilibrium [12]. The clinical technique of alveolar corticotomy and orthodontic tooth movement is unique in that periodontal tissues intentionally wounded cannot completely repair until the tooth movement stops. The only other technique similar in man is distraction osteogenesis and its periodontal equivalent, dental distraction [71]. If a subclinical wounding technique (orthodontic tooth movement) is superimposed upon an intentional surgical wounding technique (alveolar corticotomy), the repair processes surrounding the moving teeth are functioning appropriate to tissue strains ~3000–8000 με and this is a microenvironment of trabecular bone modeling and woven bone. Following any significant injury, bone strength immediately decreases and the space that is occupied by woven bone becomes maximized at about 7 days after the injury. However, between 7 and 14 days, bone strength nearly doubles and presurgical bone strength is reattained due to the rapid mineralization of woven bone [138]. Teeth moving during woven bone formation will be more rapid than teeth moving during lamellar bone formation because woven bone is hypomineralized, and as long as the teeth keep moving, the woven bone cannot fully mature (mineralize). After a few weeks of healing, moving teeth reach a more mineralized microenvironment and tooth movement slows to a microenvironment dictated by lamellar bone formation. This explains why the accelerated translation tooth movement lasts only 6–8 weeks in large experimental animals [14, 55, 91, 123, 124] and in humans [1].

Decortication creates greater than minimum effective micro-damage strain (>3000 με) within a viscoelastic/poroelastic environment resulting in deformation of cells and tissues and increases in intramedullary pressure. This creates a progenitor microenvironment favoring trabecular bone modeling and a woven bone response scaled to the level of initial bone damage that increases tissue strength [138]. Because trabecular bone is thin, catabolic modeling (A-R) plays the key role in demineralization. Following alveolar decortication, the trabecular bone anabolic modeling is upregulated at least two to three times greater [125]. Frost [29, 34, 35] described regional acceleratory phenomenon denoting that the exuberant local response increases strength and reduces strain. The medullary cavity microenvironment after corticotomy is richly vascularized and replete with osteoblast progenitors high in osteoid production, but the PDL prevents mineralization of the woven bone surrounding moving teeth until tooth movement ceases. By day 14 after injury, the woven bone tissue is still relatively hypomineralized compared with cortical bone, but other spectroscopic features of the mineral and collagen of 14-day woven bone are equivalent or only modestly different from mature cortical bone [138]. After teeth stop moving, the partially mineralized woven bone provides a scaffold for additional bone deposition and woven bone is eventually converted into lamellar bone [42]. Bone strength increases via anabolic modeling with lamellar bone production on subperiosteal surfaces, but the contribution of woven bone produced within the medullary space most certainly contributes the greatest amount to bone strength.

It has been proposed that orchestration of these complex series of events is beyond the cell level and is the responsibility of the intermediary organization [29].

Alveolar decortication that dramatically influences the role of an intermediary organization in orchestrating subsequent events is unknown and uninvestigated. Strain-dependent and hydrostatic pressure-dependent signaling under conditions of tooth movement following decortication with effective tissue strain levels exceeding micro-damage level (>3000 $\mu\varepsilon$) can only be surmised.

2.3 A Unifying Model: Tissue Strain

All of the mechanobiological cell-centric models for tooth movement described from the mid-2000s to present [53, 61–63, 77, 78, 82, 139, 154, 156] are assembled on reductionist data gathered on objective bodies or physiological entities through third-person methodologies [151] within the context of the prevailing pressure-tension tooth movement model. None of these tooth movement models to date reflect the lived or phenomenal body through first-person research methodologies [151], i.e., none reflect that the human body is sensitive to energy flow and that the dynamic strength changes interpreted by the musculoskeletal system is what drives the host demand to preserve mechanical and physiological competence.

None of the models proposed in orthodontic literature to date give serious consideration to the orchestrating influences of stress-induced microenvironments and to minimum effective strains [26, 30, 34, 38] that are capable of switching on and off stimulus–cell and cell–cell mechanisms. Tissue strain was discussed in these accounts as a mediating factor but it was the central role of the cells that prevailed. For example, the mechanobiological model proposed by Henneman [47] has been used to describe tooth movement in four stages after orthodontic force application oriented at the cell: (1) immediate matrix strain and fluid flow in both PDL and alveolar bone tissues; (2) cell deformation resulting from matrix strain; (3) cell activation and differentiation in response to cell deformation, i.e., fibroblasts and osteoblasts in the PDL and osteocytes in the bone; and (4) bone modeling and remodeling, i.e., apposition and resorption, enabling tooth movement. Likewise, the mechanobiological model proposed by Van Schepdael et al. [139] predicted tooth movement based on the activity of PDL cells by considering nine coupled nonlinear partial differential equations and two distinct signaling pathway. The molecular biological account for accelerated tooth movement proposed by Huang [53] likewise reverts to the cell-centric, compression-tension orientation with some mention of tissue strain and fluid flow.

It has been made clear during the past 15 years that physical factors beyond orthodontic loads such as corticotomy surgery may be used to improve or accelerate tissue turnover and accelerate tooth movement. Mechanical stimuli whether it be stretch, compression, pressure, or enhanced perfusion/transport can greatly enhance matrix formation in the context of tissue engineering [43]. Alveolar decortication as a functional tissue engineering technique forces attention to which mechanobiological properties are the most important in understanding of tooth movement in both native and repair tissues. And it is clear that catabolic and anabolic modeling of trabecular bone is the number one priority activity in tooth movement with and without accelerated orthodontic technique.

Native tissues are in-and-of-themselves complex in architecture and behavior. Functional tissue engineering techniques such as alveolar decortication show that repair tissues experience an altered mechanical environment. Compared to native tissues, there is an upregulation of activity and physiology as well as differences in mechanical properties. Superimposing engineered tissue repair onto tooth movement introduces time- and spatially varying stresses, strains, fluid pressure, fluid flow, and other biophysical parameters [43]. Knowledge of the mechanobiological context in which normal and repair tissues strive for homeostasis is essential, and that context is the range and history of stresses and strains placed on tissues and a thorough understanding of mechanical "thresholds" [34]. Orthopedist Harold Frost [27] was the first to articulate the importance of functional bone strain as a controlling stimulus for bone architecture, a relationship that has come to be known as the mechanostat [29, 31, 34, 59, 132]. Those adapting Frost's mechanostat to orthodontics by portraying the concept graphically were Melsen [84], Roberts [112, 115], Tyrovola [136], and Verna [142].

Host tissues are strain dependent. Response to tissue strain is aimed at preserving load-bearing structural integrity and physiological competence of skeletal tissues so signaling for bone modeling is likely turned on because increased bone strength is needed to reduce future strain demands on the skeleton [36, 87]. The prime objective of bone's adaptive modeling and remodeling activities is to produce a mass and arrangement of bone tissue in which functional loads produce strains that are appropriate in both their distribution and magnitude [118]. The biologic "machinery" that determines skeletal strength forms a tissue-level negative feedback system and monitors bone metabolism [29, 38]. These signals give rise to sophisticated and distinct biomechanical and biophysical environments at the pericellular (microscopic) and collagen/mineral molecular (nanoscopic) levels, which are the direct stimulations that positively influence bone adaptation [110].

Tissue strain concept is a unifying concept that is posited for the lived body wherein host tissues are governed by minimum effective strain levels that account for individual variation. In the context of orthodontic tooth movement, bone modeling is the dominant adaptive response to increased loads and the changes in tissue strains and intramedullary hydrostatic pressures resulting [132]. Even the slightest of strain increases produce an adaptive response in which bone apposition occurs practically unaccompanied by bone resorption [118]. It is postulated that strain-centered anabolic and catabolic modeling are the predominate characteristics of orthodontic tooth movement. Sugiyama et al. [132] suggests that bone mass/strength increases in a progressive, essentially linear relation with increasing strain-related stimulus derived from functional loading (Fig. 2.2). Where dynamic strains exceed a minimum effective skeletal modeling threshold range, mechanically controlled modeling turns on [132] to increase the local strength and reduce later strains (Fig. 2.2); adaptive modeling increases strength by adding more tissue and/or changing a structure's micro- or macro-architecture [29, 30, 36].

Orthodontic tooth movement probably induces alveolar bone strains ranging from about 1500 to 3000 $\mu\varepsilon$ and would be generally within the adaptive-mild overload or physiologic range. Alveolar corticotomy surgery most assuredly induces

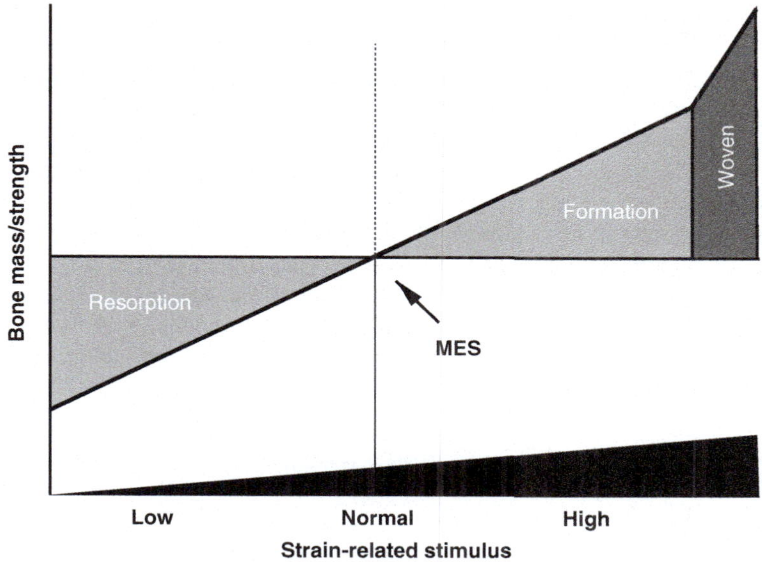

Fig. 2.2 A schematic diagram illustrating the progressive, essentially linear increase in bone mass/strength with increasing strain-related stimulus derived from functional load-bearing. In a bone that has already adapted to any level of load-bearing, any increase or decrease in strain-related stimulus will be associated with an increase or a decrease, respectively, in bone mass/strength. At one extreme, bone loss will continue until a genetically determined minimum level is achieved. At the other extreme, the osteogenic response to loading will involve exuberant woven bone formation. This level of strain will probably be associated with increased levels of micro-damage. *MES* minimum effective strain (From Sugiyama et al. [132])

strain conditions exceeding the minimum effective micro-damage or overload threshold range, i.e., >3000 $\mu\varepsilon$ (Fig. 2.1). It is surmised that high strain levels post corticotomy surgery supersede tooth movement strain levels and therefore becomes the prevailing strain-directing mechanobiological activity. The cellular response to orthodontic force after alveolar corticotomy is categorically different because the PDL and osseous microenvironments, with and without decortication surgery, differ substantially. When bone strain is high (>3000 $\mu\varepsilon$), bone mass and strength gains need to be high and swift. Woven bone production, in contrast to lamellar bone production, provides the greatest osteogenic gain and signifies response to high strain in the micro-damage range [73, 131]. Alveolar bone injury acquired by decortication certainly triggers a woven bone response that leads to a functional repair of whole-bone strength, and the woven bone response is damage-dependent, i.e., woven bone increases with increasing damage [73, 131].

The tissue strain-dependent hypothesis is that orthodontic appliance forces will be sensed as quantum energy and mechanical signals related to bone strength at various intermediary organization levels which will stimulate the guiding influences for micro- and nano-environment adaptation. In the beagle dog force threshold case described above, the superimposition or decortication surgery and tissue strains exceeding micro-damage strain threshold (>3000 με) would create a microenvironment that supersedes the tissue strain influences of tooth movement (1500–3000 με). Tooth movement adjacent to the decortication is rapid [1, 14, 55, 91, 123, 124] because demineralization of trabecular bone is rapid as is the production of woven bone which does not impede accelerated tooth movement as long as teeth are moving and the osteoid cannot mineralize. The mechanical strain and hydrostatic pressure created from the surgical wounding affects tissues of the PDL and beyond; the greater the amount and/or magnitude of the surgery, the greater the area influenced. Whole-bone strain following decortication perceived in the micro-damage threshold range creates RAP [38, 70, 142] and potentiates modeling of the trabecular bone; all metabolic activities within that region will be affected including the PDL and tooth movement (Table 2.1).

Table 2.1 Relationship between the strain-dependent theory and orthodontics-only and orthodontics + alveolar decortication

	Strain-dependent tissue influences and guiding at intermediary bone level			
	Periodontal ligament space		Medullary cavity	
Ortho load	Ortho only (1–2 Kμε modeling strain and lamellar apposition)	Ortho + decort (3–8 Kμε micro-damage strain and woven bone created)	Ortho only (1–2 Kμε modeling strain and lamellar apposition)	Ortho + decort (3–8 Kμε micro-damage strain and woven bone created)
Initial	Compressed .3 mm; ischemia	Compressed .3 mm; angiogenesis	Steady state	RAP; increased cellular activity
1 week	.3 mm TM; hyalinization	1 mm TM; RAP; angiogenesis	Mostly steady state; initial lamina dura undermining resorption	RAP; angiogenesis; modeling and increased cellular activities; undermining resorption of lamina dura
2 weeks	.4 mm TM; hyalinization; macrophages	1.5 mm TM; RAP; modeling activities	Steady state; signs of lamina dura undermining resorption	RAP; extensive angiogenesis; active modeling activities; little calcified bone; no lamina dura
4 weeks	.6 mm TM; macrophages; vascularization	2 mm TM; RAP; high modeling	Noticeable undermining resorption; modeling near PDL	RAP; ample osteoid leading to woven bone; no calcified bone
6 weeks	1.3 mm TM; modeling with mineralized bone on tension side	3 mm TM; RAP	Undermining resorption; lamina dura disappears; modeling	RAP; ample woven bone beginning to calcify at sites distant from the moving tooth
Activity	Lamellar bone modeling	Woven bone modeling	Lamellar bone modeling	Woven bone modeling

A seminal orthodontic article entitled, in part, *Biology of Biomechanics*, was recently published reflecting a physics-over-biology point of view [116]. Finite element analysis (FEA) was used to model en masse retraction of the mandibular arch in the conservative treatment of a skeletal Class III malocclusion. It was concluded that instantaneous FEA, as modeled in the article, could be used to reasonably predict the clinical results of an applied orthodontic load. The FEA formulation using a priori strain levels as best understood within the PDL at rest does not, however, account for the variations from individual to individual or the dynamic spatiotemporal changes in load variations or vacillations in tissue strain levels during adaptation. The lead author, following a lifetime of research on the dynamics of orthodontic tooth movement, adroitly points out that measuring tissue strain is simply not reliable, possible, or practical and that the appropriate, noninvasive tissue strain measuring technology has simply not evolved. The reverse engineering approach, represented in the *Biology of Biomechanics*, is a conceptual breakthrough but still does not explain the observations of inter-patient variability or adequately explain the experimental data sets and observations made in the multitude of clinical orthodontic articles. Perhaps a tissue strain-centric model for tooth movement mechanobiology is a holy grail – but it is a unifying concept worth pursuing.

References

1. Aboul-Ela SM, El-Beialy AR, El-Sayed KM, Selim EM, El-Mangoury NH, Mostafa YA. Miniscrew implant-supported maxillary canine retraction with and without corticotomy facilitated orthodontics. Am J Orthod Dentofacial Orthop. 2011;139:252–9.
2. Alikhani M, Alyami B, Lee IS, Almoammar S, Vongthongleur T, Alansari S, Sangsuwon C, Chou MY. Saturation of the biological response to orthodontic forces and its effect on the rate of tooth movement. Orthod Craniofac Res. 2015;18 Suppl 1:8–17.
3. Arwert EN, Hoste E, Watt FM. Epithelial stem cells, wound healing and cancer. Nat Rev Cancer. 2012;12:170–80.
4. Bala Y, Farley D, Delmas PD, Meunier PJ, Boivin G. Time sequence of secondary mineralization and microhardness in cortical and cancellous bone from ewes. Bone. 2010; 46:1204–12.
5. Betts DC, Muller R. Mechanical regulation of bone regeneration: theories, models, and experiments. Front Endocrinol (Lausanne). 2014;5:1–14.
6. Birmingham E, Grogan JA, Niebur GL, McNamara LM, McHugh PE. Computational modelling of the mechanics of trabecular bone and marrow using fluid structure interaction techniques. Ann Biomed Eng. 2013;41:814–26.
7. Boivin G, Bala Y, Doublier A, Farley D, Ste-Marie LG, Meunier PJ, Delmas PD. The role of mineralization and organic matrix in the microhardness of bone tissue from controls and osteoporotic patients. Bone. 2008;43:532–8.
8. Burr DB, Schaffler MB, Yang KH, Lukoschek M, Kandzari D, Sivaneri N, Blaha JD, Radin EL. The effects of altered strain environments on bone tissue kinetics. Bone. 1989; 10:223–33.
9. Burr DB, Schaffler MB, Yang KH, Lukoschek M, Sivaneri N, Blaha JD, Radin EL. Skeletal change in response to altered strain environments: Is woven bone a response to elevated strain? Bone. 1989;10:223–33.
10. Buschang PH, Campbell PM, Ruso S. Accelerating tooth movement with corticotomies: is it possible and desirable? Semin Orthod. 2012;18:286–94.

11. Carel H. Phenomenology and its application in medicine. Theor Med Bioeth. 2011;32: 33–46.
12. Chen F-M, Zhang J, Zhang M, An Y, Chen F, Wu Z-F. A review on endogenous regenerative technology in periodontal regenerative medicine. Biomaterials. 2010;31:7892–927.
13. Chen X, Li N, Yang L, Liu J, Chen J, Liu H. Expression of collagen I, collagen III and MMP-1 on the tension side of distracted tooth using periodontal ligament distraction osteogenesis in beagle dogs. Arch Oral Biol. 2014;59:1217–25.
14. Cho KW, Cho SW, Oh CO, Ryu YK, Ohshima H, Jung HS. The effect of cortical activation on orthodontic tooth movement. Oral Dis. 2007;13:314–9.
15. Chow JW, Jagger CJ, Chambers TJ. Characterization of osteogenic response to mechanical stimulation in cancellous bone of rat caudal vertebrae. Am J Physiol. 1993;265:E340–7.
16. Chow JWM, Wilson AJ, Chambers TJ, Fox SW. Mechanical loading stimulates bone formation by reactivation of bone lining cells in 13-week-old rats. J Bone Miner Res. 1998;13:1760–7.
17. Clements CD. Bioethical essentialism and scientific population thinking. Perspect Biol Med. 1985;28(2):188–207.
18. Comiskey P, MacDonald BJ, McCartney WT, Synnott K, O'Byrne J. The role of interfragmentary strain on the rate of bone healing—a new interpretation and mathematical model. J Biomech. 2010;43:2830–4.
19. Cowin SC, Cardoso L. Blood and interstitial flow in the hierarchical pore space architecture of bone tissue. J Biomech. 2015;48:842–54.
20. Curry JD. The many adaptations of bone. J Biomech. 2003;36:1487–95.
21. Davidovitch Z. Tooth movement. Crit Rev Oral Biol Med. 1991;2(4):411–50.
22. de Jong JJA, Willems PC, Arts JJ, Bours SGP, Brink PRG, van Geel TACM, Poeze M, Geusens PP, van Rietbergen B, van den Bergh JPW. Assessment of the healing process in distal radius fractures by high resolution peripheral quantitative computed tomography. Bone. 2014;64:65–74.
23. Deguchi T, Mori M. Histochemical observations on oxidative enzymes in periodontal tissue during experimental tooth movement in rat. Arch Oral Biol. 1968;13:49–59.
24. Doblaré M, Garcıa JM, Gomez MJ. Modelling bone tissue fracture and healing: a review. Eng Fract Mech. 2004;71:1809–40.
25. Eyckmans J, Boudou T, Yu X, Chen CS. A hitchhiker's guide to mechanobiology. Dev Cell. 2011;21:35–47.
26. (Editorial – No authors listed). Spatiotemporal mechanisms of life (editorial). Nat Chem Biol. 2007;3(10):593. doi:10.1038/nchembio1007-593.
27. Frost HM. Mathematical elements of lamellar bone remodeling. Springfield: IL CC Thomas; 1964.
28. Frost HM. Mechanical determinants of bone modeling. Metab Bone Dis Relat Res. 1982;4: 217–29.
29. Frost HM. The skeletal intermediary organization. Metab Bone Dis Relat Res. 1983;4: 281–90.
30. Frost HM. The "new bone": some anthropological potentials. Am J Phys Antrhr. 1985;28(S6): 211–26.
31. Frost HM. Bone "mass" and the "mechanostat": a proposal. Anat Rec. 1987;219:1–9.
32. Frost HM. The biology of fracture healing. An overview for clinicians. Part I. Clin Orthop Relat Res. 1989;248:283–93.
33. Frost HM. The biology of fracture healing. An overview for clinicians. Part II. Clin Orthop Relat Res. 1989;248:294–309.
34. Frost HM. Perspectives: bone's mechanical usage windows. Bone Miner. 1992;19: 257–71.
35. Frost HM. The Utah paradigm of skeletal physiology: an overview of its insights for bone, cartilage and collagenous tissue organs. J Bone Miner Metab. 2000;18:305–16.
36. Frost HM. Why should many skeletal scientists and clinicians learn the Utah paradigm of skeletal physiology? J Musculoskelet Neuronal Interact. 2001;2(2):121–30.

37. Frost HM. Bone's mechanostat: a 2003 update. Anat Rec A Discov Mol Cell Evol Biol. 2003;275A:1081–101.
38. Frost HM. A 2003 update of bone physiology and Wolff's Law for clinicians. Angle Orthod. 2004;74:3–15.
39. Garant PR, Cho MI. Cytoplasmic polarization of periodontal ligament fibroblasts. Implications for cell migration and collagen secretion. J Periodontal Res. 1979;14:95–106.
40. Generson RM, Porter JM, Zell A, Stratigos GT. Combined surgical and orthodontic management of anterior open bite using corticotomy. J Oral Surg. 1978;36:216–9.
41. Gould L, Abadir P, Brem H, et al. Chronic wound repair and healing in older adults: current status and future research. J Am Geriatr Soc. 2015;63:427–38.
42. Greenstein G, Greenstein B, Cavallaro J, Tarnow D. The role of bone decortication in enhancing the results of guided bone regeneration: a literature review. J Periodontol. 2009;80:175–89.
43. Guilak F, Butler DL, Goldstein SA, Baaijens FPT. Biomechanics and mechanobiology in functional tissue engineering. J Biomech. 2014;47:1933–40.
44. Gurtner GC, Werner S, Barrandon Y, Longaker MT. Wound repair and regeneration. Nature. 2008;453:314–21.
45. Hambli R. Connecting mechanics and bone cell activities in the bone remodeling process: an integrated finite element modeling. Front Bioeng Biotechnol. 2014;2:6. doi:10.3389/fbioe.2014.00006.
46. Hanley M. Naturalizing phenomenology – a philosophical imperative. Prog Biophys Mol Biol. 2015;119:661–9.
47. Henneman S, Von den Hoff JW, Maltha JC. Mechanobiology of tooth movement. Eur J Orthod. 2008;30:299–306.
48. Hillsley MV, Frangos JA. Bone tissue engineering: the role of interstitial fluid flow. Biotechnol Bioeng. 1994;43:573–81.
49. Howard PS, Kucich U, Taliwal R, Korostoff JM. Mechanical forces alter extracellular matrix synthesis by human periodontal ligament fibroblasts. J Periodontal Res. 1998;33:500–8.
50. Hu M, Cheng J, Qin YX. Dynamic hydraulic flow stimulation on mitigation of trabecular bone loss in a rat functional disuse model. Bone. 2012;51:819–25.
51. Hu M, Tian GW, Gibbons DE, Jiao J, Qin YX. Dynamic fluid flow induced mechanobiological modulation of in situ osteocyte calcium oscillations. Arch Biochem Biophys. 2015;579:55–61.
52. Hu M, Serra-Hsu F, Bethel N, Lin L, Ferreri S, Cheng J, Qin YX. Dynamic hydraulic fluid stimulation regulated intramedullary pressure. Bone. 2013;57:137–41.
53. Huang H, Williams RC, Kyrkanides S. Accelerated orthodontic tooth movement: molecular mechanisms. Am J Orthod Dentofacial Orthop. 2014;146:620–32.
54. Hughes JM, Petit MA. Biological underpinnings of Frost's mechanostat thresholds: the important role of osteocytes. J Musculoskelet Neuronal Interact. 2010;10(2):128–35.
55. Iino S, Sakoda S, Ito G, Nishimori T, Ikeda T, Miyawaki S. Acceleration of orthodontic tooth movement by alveolar corticotomy in the dog. Am J Orthod Dentofacial Orthop. 2007;131:448.e1–8.
56. Ingber DE. Tensegrity-based mechanosensing from macro to micro. Prog Biophys Mol Biol. 2008;97:163–79.
57. Ingber DE. From cellular mechanotransduction to biologically inspired engineering. Ann Biomed Eng. 2010;38:1148–61.
58. Jacobs C, Grimm S, Ziebart T, Walter C, Wehrbein H. Osteogenic differentiation of periodontal fibroblasts is dependent on the strength of mechanical strain. Arch Oral Biol. 2013;58:896–904.
59. Jee WSS. Principles in bone physiology. J Musculoskelet Neuronal Interact. 2000;1:11–3.
60. Köle H. Surgical operation on the alveolar ridge to correct occlusal abnormalities. Oral Surg Oral Med Oral Pathol. 1959;12:515–29.
61. Krishnan V, Davidovitch Z. Cellular, molecular, and tissue-level reactions to orthodontic force. Am J Orthod Dentofacial Orthop. 2006;129:469.e1–469.e32.

62. Krishnan V, Davidovitch Z. On a path to unfolding the biological mechanisms of orthodontic tooth movement. J Dent Res. 2009;88(7):597–608.
63. Krishnan V, Davidovitch Z. Biological mechanisms of tooth movement. 2nd ed. Hoboken: Wiley-Blackwell; 2015 07030-5774.
64. Lacroix D, Prendergast PJ, Li G, March D. Biomechanical model to simulate tissue differentiation and bone regeneration: application to fracture healing. Med Biol Eng Comput. 2002;40:14–21.
65. Lambers FM, Koch K, Kuhn G, Ruffoni D, Weigt C, Schulte FA, Müller R. Trabecular bone adapts to long-term cyclic loading by increasing stiffness and normalization of dynamic morphometric rates. Bone. 2013;55:325–34.
66. Lee W, Karapetyan G, Moats R, Yamashita DD, Moon HB, Ferguson DJ, et al. Corticotomy-/osteotomy-assisted tooth movement micro-CTs differ. J Dent Res. 2008;87:861–7.
67. Letechipia JE, Alessi A, Rodriguez G, Asbun J. Would increased interstitial fluid flow through in situ mechanical stimulation enhance bone remodeling? Med Hypotheses. 2010;75:196–8.
68. Leung DYM, Glagov S, Mathews MA. A new in vitro system for studying cell response to mechanical stimulation. Exp Cell Res. 1977;109:285–98.
69. Li M, Zhao Y, Hao H, Han W, Fu X. Mesenchymal stem cell–based therapy for nonhealing wounds: today and tomorrow. Wound Repair Regen. 2015. doi:10.1111/wrr.12304.
70. Liem AML, Hoogeveen EJ, Jansma J, Ren Y. Surgically facilitated experimental movement of teeth: systematic review. Br J Oral Maxillofac Surg. 2015;53:491–506.
71. Liou EJW, Huang CS. Rapid canine retraction through distraction of the periodontal ligament. Am J Orthod Dentofacial Orthop. 1998;114:372–82.
72. Love AC. Typology reconfigured: from the metaphysics of essentialism to the epistemology of representation. Acta Biotheor. 2009;57:51–75.
73. Lynch AJ, Silva MJ. In vivo static creep loading of the rat forelimb reduces ulnar structural properties at time-zero and induces damage-dependent woven bone formation. Bone. 2008;42:942–9.
74. Manjubala I, Liu Y, Epari DR, Roschger P, Schell H, Fratzl P, Duda GN. Spatial and temporal variations of mechanical properties and mineral content of the external callus during bone healing. Bone. 2009;45:185–92.
75. Martin P, Nunan R. Cellular and molecular mechanisms of repair in acute and chronic wound healing. Br J Dermatol. 2015. doi:10.1111/bjd.13954.
76. Martinez MD, Schmid GJ, Mckenzie JA, Ornitz DM, Silva MJ. Healing of non-displaced fractures produced by fatigue loading of the mouse ulna. Bone. 2010;46:1604–12.
77. Masella RS, Meister M. Current concepts in the biology of orthodontic tooth movement. Am J Orthod Dentofacial Orthop. 2006;129(4):458–68.
78. Masella RS, Chung P-L. Thinking beyond the wire: emerging biologic relationships in orthodontics and periodontology. Semin Orthod. 2008;14:290–304.
79. McBride SH, Dolejs S, Brianza S, Knothe U, Knothe Tate ML. Net change in periosteal strain during Stance shift loading after surgery correlates to rapid de novo bone generation in critically sized defects. Ann Biomed Eng. 2011;39(5):1570–81.
80. McKenzie JA, Silva MJ. Comparing histological, vascular and molecular responses associated with woven and lamellar bone formation induced by mechanical loading in the rat ulna. Bone. 2011;48:250–8.
81. Meeran NA. Biological response at the cellular level within the periodontal ligament on application of orthodontic force – an update. J Orthod Sci. 2012;1(1):2–10.
82. Meikle MC. The tissue, cellular, and molecular regulation of orthodontic tooth movement: 100 years after Carl Sandstedt. Eur J Orthod. 2006;28:221–40.
83. Melsen B. Biological reaction of alveolar bone to orthodontic tooth movement. Angle Orthod. 1999;69:151–8.
84. Melsen B. Tissue reaction to orthodontic tooth movement – a new paradigm. Eur J Orthod. 2001;23:671–81.

85. Mengoni M, Ponthot JP. An enhanced version of a bone-remodelling model based on the continuum damage mechanics theory. Comput Methods Biomech Biomed Engin. 2015;18: 1367–76.
86. Metzger TA, Schwaner SA, LaNeve AJ, Kriepke TC, Niebur GL. Pressure and shear stress in trabecular bone marrow during whole bone loading. J Biomech. 2015;48:3035–43.
87. Miller GJ, Gerstenfeld LC, Morgan EF. Mechanical microenvironments and protein expression associated with formation of different skeletal tissues during bone healing. Biomech Model Mechanobiol. 2015. doi:10.1007/s10237-015-0670-4.
88. Milne TJ, Ichim I, Patel B, McNaughton A, Meikle MC. Induction of osteopenia during experimental tooth movement in the rat: alveolar bone remodelling and the mechanostat theory. Eur J Orthod. 2009;31:221–31.
89. Mohamed AM. An overview of bone cells and their regulating factors of differentiation. Malays J Med Sci. 2008;15:4–12.
90. Morgan EF, Yeh OC, Keaveny TM. Damage in trabecular bone at small strains. Eur J Morphol. 2005;42:13–21.
91. Mostafa YA, Fayed MM, Mehanni S, ElBokle NN, Heider AM. Comparison of corticotomy-facilitated vs standard tooth movement techniques in dogs with miniscrews as anchor units. Am J Orthod Dentofacial Orthop. 2009;136:570–7.
92. Murphy N, Wilcko MT, Wilcko WM, Ferguson DJ. Periodontal accelerated osteogenic orthodontics: a description of the surgical technique. J Oral Maxillofac Surg. 2009;67: 2160–6.
93. Nanci A, Bosshardt DD. Structure of periodontal tissues in health and disease. Periodontol 2000. 2006;40:11–28.
94. Natali AN, Pavana PG, Venturatoa C, Komatsub K. Constitutive modeling of the non-linear visco-elasticity of the periodontal ligament. Comput Methods Programs Biomed. 2011;104:193–8.
95. Nie J, Fu X, Han W. Microenvironment-dependent homeostasis and differentiation of epidermal basal undifferentiated keratinocytes and their clinical applications in skin repair. J Eur Acad Dermatol Venereol. 2012;27:531–5.
96. Oppenheim A. Tissue changes, particularly of the bone, incident to tooth movement. Trans Eur Orthodont Soc. 1911;8:303–59.
97. Owan I, Burr DB, Turner CH, Qiu J, Tu Y, Onyia JE, Duncan RL. Mechanotransduction in bone: osteoblasts are more responsive to fluid forces than mechanical strain. Am J Physiol. 1997;273:C810–5.
98. Ozaki S, Kaneko S, Podyma-Inoue KA, Yanagishita M, Soma K. Modulation of extracellular matrix synthesis and alkaline phosphatase activity of periodontal ligament cells by mechanical stress. J Periodontal Res. 2005;40:110–7.
99. Papadopoulou K, Hasan I, Keilig L, Reimann S, Eliades T, Jäger A, Deschner J, Bourauel C. Biomechanical time dependency of the periodontal ligament: a combined experimental and numerical approach. Eur J Orthod. 2013;35:811–8.
100. Parfitt AM. Quantum concept of bone remodeling and turnover: implications for the pathogenesis of osteoporosis. Calcif Tissue Int. 1979;28:1–5.
101. Pilon JJGM, Kuijpers-Jagtman AM, Maltha JC. Magnitude of orthodontic forces and rate of bodily tooth movement. An experimental study. Am J Orthod Dentofacial Orthop. 1996;110:16–23.
102. Persson M. A 100th anniversary: Sandstedt's experiments on tissue changes during tooth movement. J Orthod. 2005;32:27–8.
103. Polimeni G, Xiropaidis AV, Wikesjo UME. Biology and principles of periodontal wound healing/regeneration. Periodontol 2000. 2006;41:30–47.
104. Polverini PJ. The pathophysiology of angiogenesis. Crit Rev Oral Biol Med. 1995;6:230–47.
105. Proffit WR, Fields HW, Sarver DM, Ackerman JL. Contemporary orthodontics. 5th ed. St. Louis: Elsevier Mosby; 2013.

106. Qin YX, Hu M. Mechanotransduction in musculoskeletal tissue regeneration: effects of fluid flow, loading, and cellular-molecular pathways. Biomed Res Int. 2014;2014:1–12.
107. Quinn RS, Yoshikawa K. A reassessment of force magnitude in orthodontics. Am J Orthod. 1985;88:252–60.
108. Raggatt LJ, Partridge NC. Cellular and molecular mechanisms of bone remodeling. J Biol Chem. 2010;285(33):25103–8.
109. Reitan K. The initial tissue reaction incident to orthodontic tooth movement as related to the influence of function. Acta Odontol Scand Suppl. 1951;6:1–240.
110. Ren J, Yang P, Wang Z, Zhang J, Ding C, Shang P. Biomechanical and biophysical environment of bone from the macroscopic to the pericellular and molecular level. J Mech Behav Biomed Mater. 2015;50:104–22.
111. Roberts WE, Chase DC. Kinetics of cell proliferation and migration associated with orthodontically-induced osteogenesis. J Dent Res. 1981;60:174–81.
112. Roberts WE, Huja A, Roberts JA. Bone modeling: biomechanics, molecular mechanisms, and clinical perspectives. Semin Orthod. 2004;10:129–42.
113. Roberts WE, Roberts JA, Epker BN, Burr DB, Hartsfield Jr JK. Remodeling of mineralized tissues, part I: the frost legacy. Semin Orthod. 2006;12:216–37.
114. Roberts WE, Roberts JA, Epker BN, Burr DB, Hartsfield Jr JK. Remodeling of mineralized tissues, part II: control and pathophysiology. Semin Orthod. 2006;12:238–53.
115. Roberts WE. Bone physiology, metabolism and biomechanics in orthodontic practice. In: Graber LW, Vanarsdall Jr RL, Vig KW, editors. Orthodontics: current principles and techniques. 5th ed. St Louis: Elsevier-Mosby; 2012. p. 287–343.
116. Roberts WE, Viecilli RF, Chang C, Katona TR, Paydare NH. Biology of biomechanics: finite element analysis of a statically determinate system to rotate the occlusal plane for correction of a skeletal class III open-bite malocclusion. Am J Orthod Dentofacial Orthop. 2015;148: 943–55.
117. Rosen SM. Why natural science needs phenomenological philosophy. Prog Biophys Mol Biol. 2015;119:257–69.
118. Rubin CT, Lanyon LE. Regulation of bone mass by mechanical strain magnitude. Calcif Tissue Int. 1985;37:411–7.
119. Rygh P, Selvig KA. Erythrocytic crystallization in rat molar periodontium incident to tooth movement. Scand J Dent Res. 1973;81:62–73.
120. Salomon E, Cimpian A. The inherence heuristic as a source of essentialist thought. Pers Soc Psychol Bulletin. 2014;40(10):1297–315.
121. Sandy JR, Farndale RW, Meikle MC. Recent advances in understanding mechanically induced bone remodeling and their relevance to orthodontic theory and practice. Am J Orthod Dentofacial Orthop. 1993;103:212–23.
122. Sandstedt C. Einige Beiträge zur Theorie der Zahnregulierung. Nord Tand Tidskr. 1904;5:236–56; 1905;6:1–25; 6:141–68.
123. Sanjideh PA, Rossouw PE, Campbell PM, Opperman LA, Buschang PH. Tooth movements in foxhounds after one or two alveolar corticotomies. Eur J Orthod. 2010;32:106–13.
124. Safavi SM, Heidarpour M, Izadi SS, et al. Effects of flapless bur decortications on movement velocity of dogs' teeth. J Dent Res. 2012;9:783–9.
125. Sebaoun JD, Turner JW, Kantarci A, Carvalho RS, Van Dyke TE, Ferguson DJ. Modeling of trabecular bone and lamina dura following selective alveolar decortication in rats. J Periodontol. 2008;79:1679–88.
126. Sims NA, Martin TJ, Coupling the activities of bone formation and resorption: a multitude of signals within the basic multicellular unit. Bonekey Rep. 2014;3(article 481):1–10.
127. Shaw TJ, Martin P. Wound repair at a glance. J Cell Sci. 2009;122:3209–13.
128. Shimono M, Ishikawa T, Ishikawa H, Matsuzaki H, Hasimoto S, Muramatsu T, Shima K, Matsuzaka K-I, Inoue T. Regulatory mechanisms of periodontal regeneration. Microsc Res Tech. 2003;60:491–502.
129. Storey E, Smith R. Force in orthodontics and its relation to tooth movement. Aust J Dent. 1952;56:11–8.

130. Suárez-Díaz E. That 70s show: regulation, evolution and development beyond molecular genetics. Hist Philos Life Sci. 2015;36(4):503–24.
131. Sugiyama T, Price JS, Lanyon LE. Functional adaptation to mechanical loading in both cortical and cancellous bone is controlled locally and is confined to the loaded bones. Bone. 2010;46:314–21.
132. Sugiyama T, Meakin LB, Browne WJ, Galea GL, Price JS, Lanyon LE. Bones' adaptive response to mechanical loading is essentially linear between the low strains associated with disuse and the high strains associated with the lamellar/woven bone transition. J Bone Miner Res. 2012;27:1784–93.
133. Temple DH, Goodman AH. Bioarcheology has a "health" problem: conceptualizing "stress" and "health" in bioarcheological research. Am J Phys Anthropol. 2014;155:186–91.
134. Turner CH, Akhter MP, Raab DM, Kiummel DB, Recker RR. A noninvasive, in vivo model for studying strain adaptive bone modeling. Bone. 1991;12:73–9.
135. Turner CH, Warden SJ, Bellido T, Plotkin LI, Kumar N, Jasiuk I, Danzig J, Robling AG. Mechanobiology of the skeleton. Sci Signal. 2009;2:1–4.
136. Tyrovola JB. The 'mechanostat theory' of frost and the OPG/RANKL/RANK system. J Cell Biochem. 2015. doi:10.1002/jcb.25265.
137. Uitto V-J. Extracellular matrix molecules and their receptors: an overview with special emphasis on periodontal tissues. Crit Rev Oral Biol Med. 1991;2:323–54.
138. Uthgenannt BA, Kramer MH, Hwu JA, Wopenka B, Silva MJ. Skeletal self-repair: stress fracture healing by rapid formation and densification of woven bone. J Bone Miner Res. 2007;22:1548–56.
139. Van Schepdael A, Vander Sloten J, Geris L. A mechanobiological model of orthodontic tooth movement. Biomech Model Mechanobiol. 2013;12:249–65.
140. van Leeuwen EJ, Kuijpers AM, Von den Hoff JW, Wagener FADTG, Maltha JC. Rate of orthodontic tooth movement after changing the force magnitude: an experimental study in beagle dogs. Orthod Craniofac Res. 2010;13:238–45.
141. Vetter A, Witt F, Sander O, Duda GN, Weinkamer R. The spatio-temporal arrangement of different tissues during bone healing as a result of simple mechanobiological rules. Biomech Model Mechanobiol. 2012;11:147–60.
142. Verna C. Regional acceleratory phenomena. In: Kantarci A, Will L, Yen S, editors. Tooth movement, Frontiers of oral biology, vol. 18. Basel: Karger; 2016. p. 28–35.
143. Verna C, Dalstra M, Melsen B. The rate and the type of orthodontic tooth movement is influenced by bone turnover in a rat model. Eur J Orthod. 2000;22:343–52.
144. Verna C, Melsen B. Tissue reaction to orthodontic tooth movement in different bone turnover. conditions. Orthod Craniofac Res. 2003;6:155–63.
145. Vodovotz Y, Constantine G, Faeder J, Mi Q, Rubin J, Bartels J, Sarkar J, Squires RH, Okonkwo DO, Gerlach J, Zamora R, Luchart S, Ermentrout B, An G. Translational systems approaches to the biology of inflammation and healing. Immunopharmacol Immunotoxicol. 2010;32:181–95.
146. Von Bohl M, Maltha J, Von den Hoff H, Kuijpers-Jagtman AM. Changes in the periodontal ligament after experimental tooth movement using high and low continuous forces in beagle dogs. Angle Orthod. 2004;74:16–25.
147. Von den Hoff JW. Effects of mechanical tension on matrix degradation by human periodontal ligament cells cultured in collagen gels. J Periodontal Res. 2003;38:449–57.
148. Warden SJ. Breaking the rules for bone adaptation to mechanical loading. J Appl Physiol. 2006;100:1441–2.
149. Webster D, Schulte FA, Lambers FM, Kuhn G, Müller R. Strain energy density gradients in bone marrow predict osteoblast and osteoclast activity: a finite element study. J Biomech. 2015;48:866–74.
150. Weiss AJ, Iqbal J, Zaidi N, Mechanick JI. The skeletal subsystem as an integrative physiology paradigm. Curr Osteoporos Rep. 2010;8:168–77.
151. Whitehead PM. Overcoming parallelism: naturalizing phenomenology with Goldstein and merleau-ponty. Prog Biophys Mol Biol. 2015;119:502–9.

152. Wilcko WM, Wilcko MT, Bouquot JE, Ferguson DJ. Rapid orthodontics with alveolar reshaping: two case reports of decrowding. Int J Periodontics Restorative Dent. 2001;21:9–19.
153. Wilcko MT, Wilcko WM, Pulver JJ, Bissada NF, Bouquot JE. Accelerated osteogenic orthodontics technique: a 1-stage surgically facilitated rapid orthodontic technique with alveolar augmentation. J Oral Maxillofac Surg. 2009;67:2149–59.
154. Wise GE, King GJ. Mechanisms of tooth eruption and orthodontic tooth movement. J Dent Res. 2008;87(5):414–34.
155. Wohl GR, Towler DA, Silva MJ. Stress fracture healing: fatigue loading of the rat ulna induces upregulation in expression of osteogenic and angiogenic genes that mimic the intramembranous portion of fracture repair. Bone. 2009;44:320–30.
156. Xiao W, Wang Y, Pacios S, Li S, Graves DT. Cellular and molecular aspects of bone remodeling. In: Kantarci A, Will L, Yen S, editors. Tooth movement, Frontiers of oral biology, vol. 18. Basel: Karger; 2016. p. 9–16.

Biphasic Theory of Tooth Movement: Cytokine Expression and Rate of Tooth Movement

3

Cytokines and Rate of Tooth Movement

Mani Alikhani, Sarah Alansari, Chinapa Sangsuwon, Jeanne Nervina, and Cristina Teixeira

Abstract

Understanding the molecular and cellular events during orthodontic tooth movement can greatly impact daily orthodontic practice. Selecting the most appropriate force magnitude, knowing precise tooth movement, optimizing activation intervals, preventing side effects, and, most importantly, developing techniques that increase the rate of tooth movement are all influenced by this understanding. These events can be divided into two main phases, a

M. Alikhani (✉)
Consortium for Translational Orthodontic Research, Hoboken, NJ, USA

Forsyth Laboratories, Boston, MA, USA

Department of Developmental Biology, Harvard School of Dental Medicine, Boston, MA, USA
e-mail: mani_alikhani@hsdm.harvard.edu

S. Alansari • J. Nervina
Consortium for Translational Orthodontic Research, Hoboken, NJ, USA

Department of Orthodontics, New York University College of Dentistry, New York, NY, USA

C. Sangsuwon
Consortium for Translational Orthodontic Research, Hoboken, NJ, USA

C. Teixeira
Consortium for Translational Orthodontic Research, Hoboken, NJ, USA

Department of Orthodontics, New York University College of Dentistry, New York, NY, USA

Department of Basic Science and Craniofacial Biology, New York University College of Dentistry, New York, NY, USA

B. Shroff (ed.), *Biology of Orthodontic Tooth Movement*,
DOI 10.1007/978-3-319-26609-1_3

catabolic phase, where osteoclast-driven bone resorption determines the rate of tooth movement, and an anabolic phase, where osteoblast-driven bone formation reestablishes and maintains alveolar bone integrity of the new occlusion. These two phases are not simultaneous or independent – the catabolic phase is required and always precedes the anabolic phase. We call this biological phenomenon the *Biphasic Theory of Tooth Movement.* While cytokines play an important role in initiating the catabolic phase, interaction between osteoclasts and osteoblasts regulates the anabolic phase. Therefore, to increase the rate of tooth movement, acceleration techniques must focus first on producing higher cytokine activity and second on enhancing osteoclast and osteoblast interactions to expand the boundary of tooth movement and maintain the integrity of alveolar bone in the newly established occlusion. In this chapter, we will review the events of both catabolic and anabolic phases of treatment and how to manipulate them to enhance orthodontic outcomes.

3.1 Introduction

The foundation of orthodontics relies on stimulating the movement of teeth through alveolar bone. This movement is initiated in response to application of orthodontic forces. While this is a daily reality of any orthodontic treatment, optimizing this movement and reducing potential risk factors remain the main challenges for researchers. To address these challenges, understanding the biology of tooth movement is fundamental.

It is generally accepted that for orthodontic force to move a tooth, bone resorption should be activated to remove the bone in the compressive path of movement, while bone formation should follow on the opposite tension side of the tooth to maintain the integrity of alveolar bone. It is important to understand that the rate of bone resorption controls the rate of tooth movement, while the rate of bone formation determines the success of treatment. Based on these concepts, the biological events of orthodontic tooth movement can be divided into two main phases: a catabolic phase when bone resorption occurs and an anabolic phase when bone formation occurs.

In spite of clarity in the overall cellular and histological events of orthodontic movement, the mechanism behind these events is ambiguous. Some of the questions that remain less agreed upon include the following: How are bone resorption and formation activated in response to orthodontic forces? Are these events the direct effect of mechanical stimulation induced by orthodontic forces, or are there indirect mediators of orthodontic tooth movement? Does the periodontal ligament (PDL) play a role in controlling the rate of tooth movement? How can the catabolic and anabolic effects of orthodontic forces be increased when needed? To address these questions, a general understanding of how each type of bone cell functions is necessary.

3.2 Bone Cells and Their Role in the Biology of Tooth Movement

Three types of bone cells play a significant role in the biology of tooth movement: osteoblasts, osteocytes, and osteoclasts. Osteoblasts are mononuclear cells found along the surface of bones. They are derived from mesenchymal stem cells in the bone marrow and synthesize collagenous and non-collagenous proteins that comprise the organic bone matrix, the osteoid. Inactive osteoblasts that cover bone surfaces, particularly in the adult skeleton, are called bone lining cells. These cells are quiescent until growth factors or other anabolic stimuli induce their proliferation and differentiation into cuboidal osteoblasts. Osteoblasts are the main cells participating in the anabolic phase of orthodontic tooth movement with a limited role during catabolic phase.

Osteocytes are mature osteoblasts embedded in lacunae within the bone matrix. Although immobile, osteocytes possess exquisitely fine processes, which traverse the mineralized matrix in tunnels called canaliculi, to make contact with other osteocytes, as well as with osteoblasts residing on the bone surface. Given their preponderance in the bone, and their intricate three-dimensional network, osteocytes are key mechanosensors that recognize mechanical load and, by regulating osteoclast and osteoblast activity, reshape the bone to fit the mechanical demand.

The mechanism by which mechanical stimulation activates osteocytes is not clear. Loading of bone under physiologic condition results in strain, or deformation, in the bone matrix and the lacunae and canaliculi that surround the osteocytes. Some authors suggest that it is the magnitude of the matrix deformation (strain) that triggers bone remodeling [27]. Conversely, others argue that load itself is not the main ostoeogenic component of mechanical stimulation, but, instead, load by-products such as strain rate [29], strain distribution [36], or fluid flow [31] are the primary remodeling initiators. While this controversy remains under active investigation, there is consensus that mechanical stimulation is detected by osteocytes via fluid shear stress produced by increased fluid flow in the lacunocanalicular system and electrical strain potentials. These responses to mechanical load activate osteocytes to secrete key factors, such as prostaglandins, nitric oxide, or insulin-like growth factors (IGFs), which then activate osteoclasts and osteoblasts in a tightly synchronized biological phenomenon called bone remodeling.

While it is clear that osteocytes are critical for normal bone remodeling, the precise role they play in the biology of tooth movement is unknown. They may play a role in the catabolic phase of movement by activating osteoclasts. However, it is more probable that they play a role in the anabolic phase by coordinating osteoblast activation.

The last cell type that plays a significant role in orthodontic tooth movement is the osteoclast, which is the major bone resorbing cell. Osteoclasts are specialized monocyte/macrophage family members, formed by the fusion of numerous monocytic precursors to create giant multinucleated cells. Terminal differentiation in this lineage is characterized by the acquisition of mature phenotypic markers, such as the calcitonin receptor, tartrate-resistant acid phosphatase (TRAP), and cathepsin K, and the appearance of a ruffled border rich in proton pumps that acidify the bone surface to which the cells are attached, resulting in resorption pits.

Osteoclasts play an important role in the catabolic phase of orthodontic tooth movement. In fact, it is osteoclasts that control the rate of bone resorption and, therefore, the rate of tooth movement. However, osteoclasts do not function independently. In fact, they require signals from other cells for their precursor recruitment, maturation, activation, and targeted, site-specific bone resorption. The consequences of unregulated osteoclast activation would be catastrophic as bone resorption would proceed unchecked producing weakened bone and fractures. Consequently, osteoclasts cannot be considered the direct target of orthodontic forces. Instead, the upstream events that control osteoclast formation and activation must be the main target. We have compiled the scientific evidence to support a new *Biphasic Theory of Tooth Movement*.

3.3 Catabolic Phase of Orthodontic Tooth Movement

3.3.1 Theories on Initiation of Tooth Movement

Orthodontic forces produce different types of movement depending on the magnitude of forces and couples applied to the teeth. Each type of tooth movement causes a specific pattern of stress distribution in different areas of the PDL and alveolar bone. It is widely accepted that the areas experiencing the highest compression stresses are the ones that undergo the highest levels of osteoclastic bone resorption. During recent years, many theories have been developed to explain the initial events of orthodontic tooth movement leading to osteoclast activation in these compression sites. In general, these theories split into two camps: one proposes that bone cells (more specifically osteocytes) are the direct target of orthodontic forces (*direct view*), while the other proposes that the PDL is the key target of treatment (*indirect view*). However, there is agreement in both theories that osteoclasts are the final cells that resorb bone and, therefore, are the cells that control the rate of tooth movement.

Using the research on weight-bearing bone as the basis of the direct view hypothesis, its proponents claim that there are two mechanisms by which direct loading may activate osteocytes. In the first mechanism, when mechanical stimulation is at physiologic levels, osteocytes recognize the different components of mechanical stimulation (such as matrix deformation) and direct the bone remodeling machinery by triggering osteoclast to remove the old bone structure and rebuild new load-friendly bone by activating osteoblasts. According to this mechanism, orthodontic tooth movement can be considered a physiologic adaptation to mechanical stimulation induced by orthodontic forces. In the second mechanism, when mechanical stimulation is at higher (pathologic) load levels, microfractures appear in the matrix that are recognized by osteocytes, which then activate the remodeling machinery. In this mechanism, orthodontic tooth movement is considered a response to trauma caused by orthodontic forces.

While the osteocyte-driven bone remodeling response to physiologic or pathologic levels of forces is supported by data derived from studies of weight-bearing bones, this theory of bone remodeling in response to orthodontic forces is questionable. Experiments in long bones and alveolar bone demonstrate that at physiologic levels, osteocytes do not recognize static forces [3, 35]. This argues against considering orthodontic tooth movement a physiologic adaptation to mechanical stimulation, since orthodontic forces are mostly static rather than intermittent. Supporting this idea, the application of orthodontic forces to dental implants used as anchorage during orthodontics treatment does not induce movement of the implant.

Can orthodontic forces stimulate tooth movement by inducing microfractures in the bone? While microfractures occur in response to orthodontic forces [42], the possibility that it is the main mechanism of tooth movement is low. The fact that orthodontic force cannot move an ankylosed tooth demonstrates that microfractures are not the main triggers for tooth movement. Moreover, the relationship between force magnitude and tooth movement is not linear, and soon after applying orthodontic force, the bone remodeling rate reaches a saturation point. If microfractures are the trigger for tooth movement, one would expect higher forces should increase the rate of movement without a saturation of the response [1, 2]. It should be emphasized that while application of higher magnitude force (at the pathologic level) may damage the bone around an implant significantly to the point of implant failure, the stronger forces do not move the implant in bone. Coupled with the fact that the lower, physiologic, magnitude of force is applied during clinical orthodontics strongly suggests that microfractures are not the trigger for orthodontic tooth movement.

Supporters of the indirect view of tooth movement propose that the PDL is the primary target of orthodontic forces. Consider the impossibility of moving an ankylosed tooth, which lacks a PDL. Based on this proposal, the PDL exhibits areas of compression and tension in response to orthodontic forces. If the duration of force application is limited to a few seconds (i.e., is intermittent), the incompressible tissue fluid prevents quick displacement of the tooth within the PDL space. However, if the force on a tooth is maintained (i.e., is static, as in orthodontic treatment), the fluid is squeezed out of the PDL, providing space for tooth displacement in the socket and further compression of the PDL. The immediate result of this displacement is blood vessel constriction in the compression site. The resulting decreased blood flow would cause a decrease in nutrient and oxygen levels (hypoxia). Depending on the magnitude of pressure and blood flow impairment, some of the cells go through apoptosis, while other cells die nonspecifically, resulting in an area of necrosis that is identified histologically as the cell-free zone. It should be emphasized that apoptotic or necrotic changes are not limited to PDL cells and some of the osteoblasts and osteocytes in adjacent alveolar bone also die in response to orthodontic forces. This sequence of events leads to an aseptic, acute inflammatory response with the early release of chemokines from local cells (Fig. 3.1).

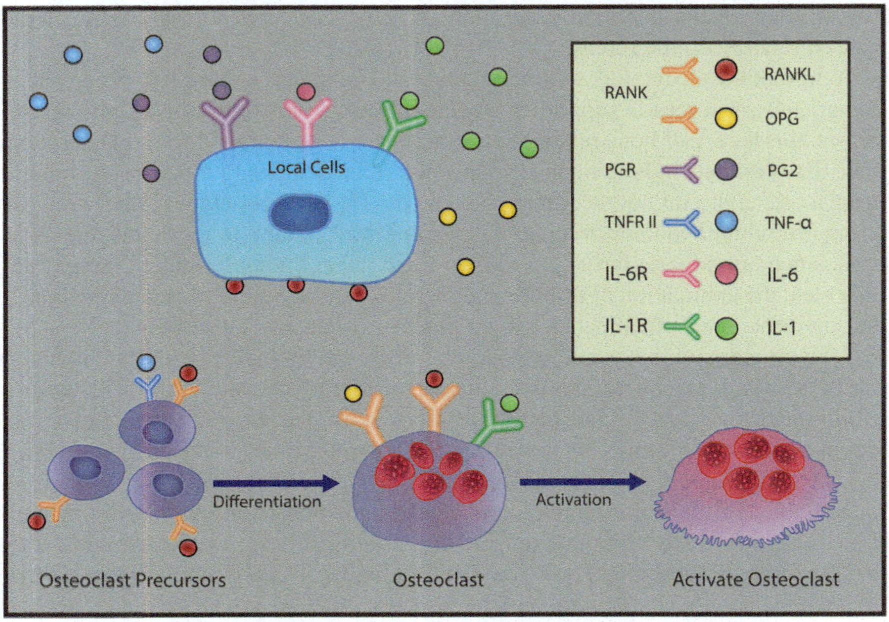

Fig. 3.1 Cytokines regulate osteoclastogenesis. Cytokines are mediators of osteoclastogenesis with important roles at different stages of this process. Some of these cytokines produced by local cells bind to receptors on the surface of osteoclast precursor cells to induce their differentiation into osteoclasts (RANKL, TNF-α), while others directly stimulate osteoclast activation (RANKL, IL1). Additionally, local cells can also downregulate osteoclastogenesis by producing a RANKL decoy receptor, osteoprotegerin (OPG)

Chemokines are small proteins released by local cells that can attract other cells to the area. The release of chemokines in response to orthodontic forces facilitates expression of adhesion molecules in blood vessels and stimulates further recruitment of inflammatory and precursor cells from the microvasculature into the extravascular space. Given their strong biological influence on localized cellular activity, it is important to discuss chemokines in the context of the biology of tooth movement and to demonstrate the role they play in our *Biphasic Theory of Tooth Movement.*

3.3.2 Initial Aseptic Inflammatory Response

One of the chemokines that is released during tooth movement is monocyte chemoattractant protein-1 (MCP-1 or CCL2) [40], which plays an important role in recruiting monocytes from the bloodstream to enter the surrounding tissue where they become tissue macrophages or, importantly to us, osteoclasts. Similarly, the release of CCL3 [9] and CCL5 (RANTES) [6] during orthodontic tooth movement leads to osteoclast recruitment and activation.

Within the first few hours of orthodontic treatment, there is further release of a broad spectrum of inflammatory mediators. Thus, in addition to chemokines, cytokines are also released during orthodontic treatment. These extracellular proteins play an important role in regulating the inflammatory process. Many cytokines are proinflammatory and help to amplify or maintain the inflammatory response and activation of bone resorption machinery. Importantly, some cytokines are anti-inflammatory, thereby preventing unrestrained progression of the inflammatory response. The main proinflammatory cytokines that are released during orthodontic tooth movement are IL-1α, IL-1β, TNF-α, and IL-6 [13]. These cytokines are produced by inflammatory cells such as macrophages and by local cells such as osteoblasts, fibroblasts, and endothelial cells.

Another series of inflammatory mediators that are released during orthodontic tooth movement are prostaglandins (PGs) and neuropeptides. PGs are derived from arachidonic acid metabolism and can mediate virtually every step of inflammation such as vasodilation, increase vascular permeability, and adhesion of inflammatory cells. During orthodontic tooth movement, these mediators can be produced directly by local cells or by inflammatory cells in response to mechanical stimulation or indirectly by cytokines. For example, TNF-α is a potent stimulator of PGE_2 formation [30]. PGs act locally at the site of generation, then decay spontaneously, or are enzymatically destroyed [11, 34]. Similar to PGs, neuropeptides can participate in many stages of the inflammatory response to orthodontic forces. Neuropeptides are small proteins, such as substance P, that transmit pain signals, regulate vessel tone, and modulate vascular permeability [24]. The importance of all these inflammatory markers can be appreciated in the role that they play in osteoclastogenesis.

3.3.3 Inflammatory Mediators Governing Osteoclastogenesis

As previously discussed, osteoclasts are multinucleated giant cells derived from hematopoietic stem cells of the monocyte-macrophage lineage that resorb bone. After recruitment to traumatized area, osteoclast precursors begin to differentiate into osteoclasts. Cytokines are important mediators of this process. For example, TNF-α and IL-1 bind to their receptors, TNFRII [12] and IL-1R [20], respectively, and directly stimulate osteoclast formation from precursor cells and osteoclast activation (Fig. 3.1). Additionally, IL-1 and IL-6 [28] can indirectly stimulate local cells or inflammatory cells to express M-CSF (macrophage colony-stimulating factor) and RANKL (receptor activator of nuclear factor B ligand). These ligands, through cell-to-cell interactions, bind to their respective receptors, c-Fms and RANK, which are both expressed on the surface of osteoclast precursors (Fig. 3.1).

Other inflammatory mediators that enhance osteoclast formation through enhancing RANKL expression by stromal cells are PGs, especially PGE_2 [39]. As mentioned before, PGs can be produced by local cells directly in response to orthodontic forces or indirectly as downstream of cytokines such as TNF-α. It should be emphasized that local cells normally downregulate osteoclastogenesis by producing a

RANKL decoy receptor, osteoprotegerin (OPG) [43]. Therefore, OPG levels in compression sites should decrease to enable tooth movement.

3.3.4 Effect of Cytokine Inhibition on the Rate of Tooth Movement

The importance of cytokines in controlling the rate of tooth movement can be appreciated from studies that block their effects. It has been shown that injection of IL-1 receptor antagonist or TNF-α receptor antagonist (sTNF-α-RI) results in a 50% reduction in tooth velocity [5, 18, 19, 22]. Similarly, tooth movement in TNF type II receptor-deficient mice is reduced compared to wild-type mice [46]. Animals deficient in chemokine receptor 2 (a receptor for chemokine ligand 2) or chemokine ligand 3 show a significant reduction in orthodontic tooth movement and the number of osteoclasts [10]. Likewise, it is well known that nonsteroidal anti-inflammatory drugs can reduce the velocity of tooth movement by inhibiting prostaglandin synthesis [8, 23]. Inhibition of other derivatives of arachidonic acid, such as leukotrienes, also significantly decreases the rate of tooth movement [26].

3.3.5 Saturation of the Biological Response

Taken together, these studies support the conclusion that inflammatory markers play a critical role in orthodontic tooth movement by controlling the rate of osteoclast formation and, therefore, bone resorption. It logically follows that increasing the magnitude of orthodontic forces would trigger a cascade of increased inflammatory marker expression and osteoclastogenesis resulting in faster tooth movement. Surprisingly, one of the biggest controversies in the biology of tooth movement literature revolves around the relation between magnitude of force and the rate of tooth movement. While some studies show that higher forces do not increase the rate of tooth movement [32, 33], others argue the opposite [44]. This paradox is explained by the inappropriate use of tooth movement as a measure of the effect of force magnitude on the rate of tooth movement. Although tooth movement is indeed the desired result of the biological response to force, it does not precisely measure the relation between force magnitude and the biological response that causes tooth movement.

Many factors affect the amount of tooth movement independent of the force magnitude. These factors can be intrinsic, such as differences in root and alveolar bone shape or bone density, or they may be extrinsic, such as occlusal forces, chewing habits, or limitation of the mechanical design. These variables are difficult to accurately assess in humans due to the need for a large group of subjects with similar anatomical features, age, gender, and type of malocclusion. While these limitations are easier to control in animal models, depending on the study duration, measuring tooth movement as the sole representative of the effect of force magnitude can still produce conflicting results because the biological response varies throughout the stages of tooth movement. Different investigators may capture different stages of this biological response and make erroneous conclusions that are not representative of the complete process.

Because of experimental design limitations mentioned above, it is more logical to study the biological response to different force magnitudes in rats that share a similar genetic background and use molecular and cellular changes, rather than the amount of tooth movement, as the outcome measurements. Recent studies demonstrate that increasing the magnitude of orthodontic force increases inflammatory marker levels, osteoclast recruitment and formation, alveolar bone resorption, and the rate of tooth movement. However, there is a force level above which we cannot stimulate these biological responses any further [1, 2]. Thus, the magnitude of cytokine release that can be induced by orthodontic forces has an upper limit, and consequently the osteoclast activity initiated by orthodontic forces has a saturation point (Fig. 3.2). While the saturation point can vary with the type of tooth movement, patient anatomy, bone density, and duration of treatment, the range of this variation is limited, and therefore, the rate of tooth movement is usually predictable. While increasing the force magnitude does not overcome this limitation, any methodology that can increase the osteoclast numbers in the area could be the answer to enhancing this biological response.

3.3.6 Effect of Cytokine Stimulation on the Rate of Tooth Movement

If inhibiting inflammatory markers decreases the rate of tooth movement, it is logical to assume that increasing their activity should significantly increase the rate of tooth movement. Indeed, injecting PGs into the PDL in rodents increases the number of osteoclasts and the rate of tooth movement [21]. Systemic application of misoprostol, a PGE_1 analog, to rats undergoing tooth movement for 2 weeks significantly increases the rate of tooth movement [38]. Similarly, local injection of other arachidonic acid derivatives, such as thromboxane and prostacyclin [15], increases the rate of tooth movement.

Another approach to increasing inflammatory mediators that can improve the rate of tooth movement is to stimulate the body to produce these factors at a higher level. The advantage of this approach is a coordinated increase in the level of all inflammatory mediators. As discussed before, many cytokines participate in response to orthodontic forces. Injecting one cytokine does not mimic the normal inflammatory response, which is a balance of pro- and anti-inflammatory mediators. However, which approach safely triggers the body to produce higher levels of inflammatory mediators is not clear.

Animal studies have shown that introducing small perforations in the alveolar bone (micro-osteoperforations (MOPs)) during orthodontic tooth movement can significantly stimulate the expression of inflammatory mediators. While application of orthodontic force beyond the saturation point does not elevate the expression and activation of inflammatory mediators beyond certain levels, adding MOPs to the

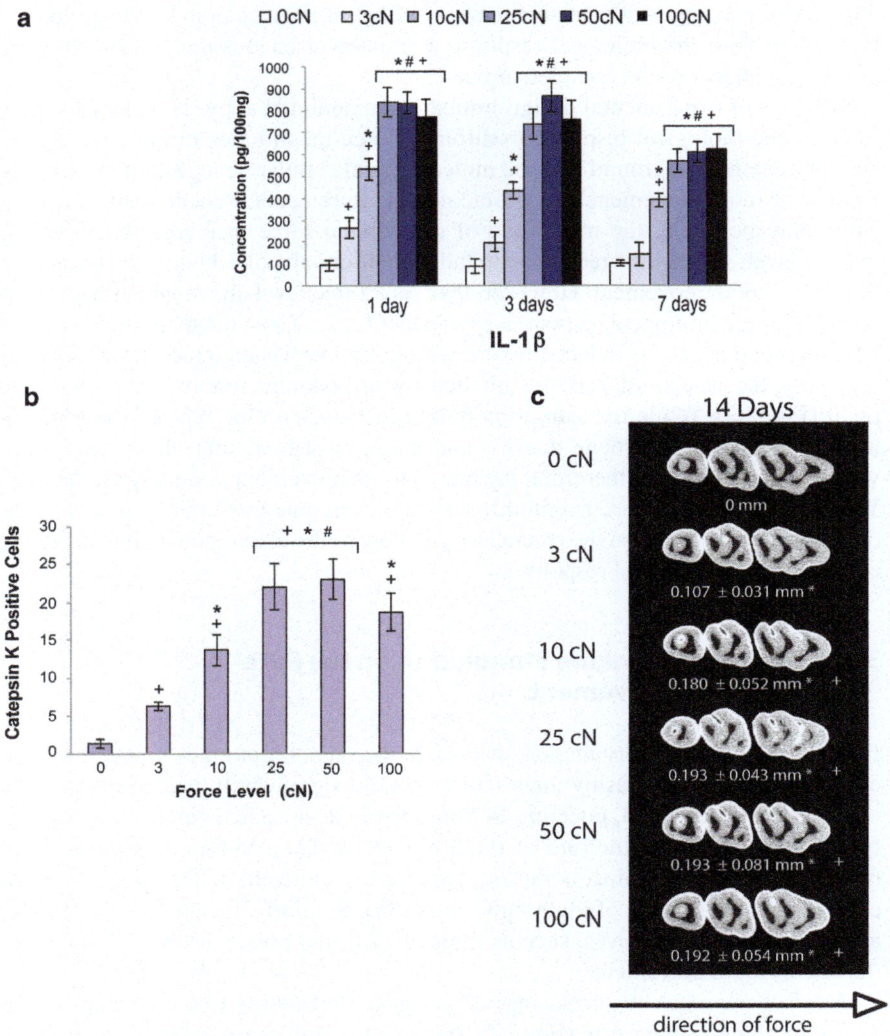

Fig. 3.2 Saturation of biological response with increased orthodontic forces. The upper right maxillary molar of rats was mesialized using different magnitude of forces (0–100 cN), and the hemimaxillae were collected for different analyses at different time points. (**a**) IL-1β was evaluated by enzyme-linked immunosorbent-based assay after 1, 3, and 7 days of force applications. Data expressed as the mean±SEM of concentration in picograms per 100 mg of tissue. (+ Significantly different from 0 cN at same time point; * significantly different from 3 cN at same time point; # significantly different from 10 cN at same time point.) (**b**) Mean numbers of osteoclasts in the PDL and adjacent alveolar bone of mesiopalatal root of maxillary molar 7 days after application of force. Osteoclasts were identified as cathepsin K-positive cells in immunohistochemical stained sections from different force groups. Each value represents the mean±SEM of five animals (+ significantly different from 0 cN; * significantly different from 3 cN; # significantly different from 10 cN). (**c**) Micro-CT images of right maxillary molars of control and different experimental groups 14 days after application of force. Each value represents the mean±SEM of the average distance between first and second molar measured at height of contour in five animals (* significantly different from 0 cN; # significantly different from 3 cN)

area of tooth movement increases the level of inflammatory mediators [41]. This response is accompanied by a significant increase in osteoclast number, bone resorption, and localized osteopenia around all adjacent teeth, which could explain the increase in the rate and magnitude of tooth movement (Fig. 3.3). One may argue that the effects of the shallow MOPs on tooth movement are not a response to increased cytokine expression, but rather due to weakening of the bone structure. While the effects that perforations can have on the physical properties of the bone cannot be ignored, the number and diameter of these perforations are too small to have

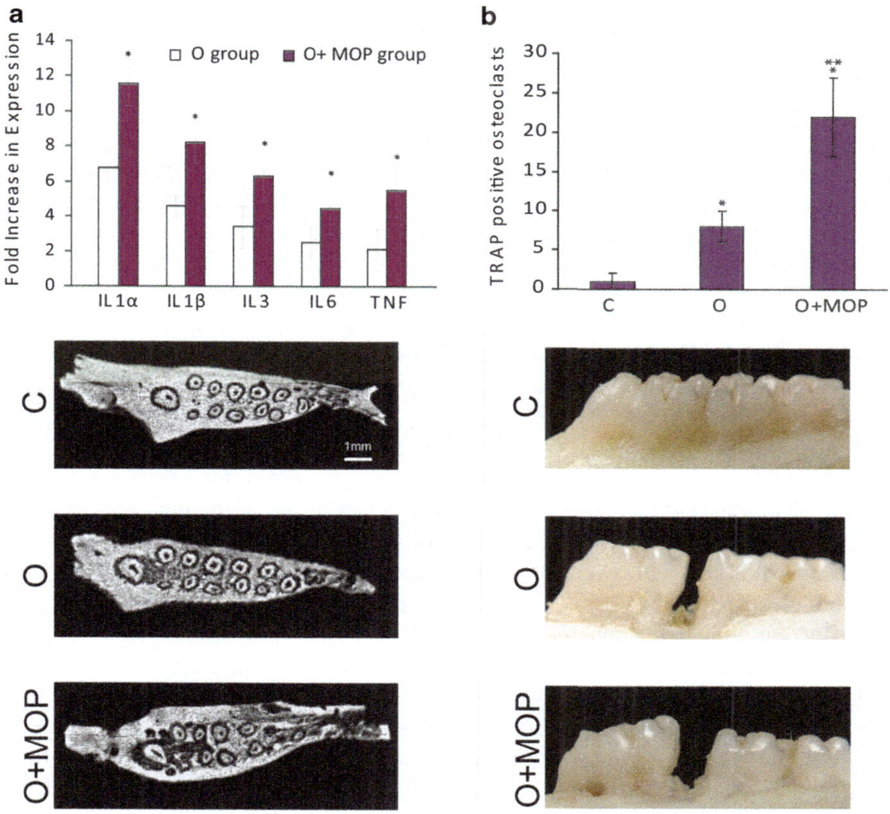

Fig. 3.3 Micro-osteoperforations increase osteoclast activity, decrease bone density, and accelerate tooth movement in rats. Rat hemimaxillae were collected 28 days after application of force to mesialize the first molar. Control group maxilla did not receive any force (*C*), O group maxilla received force only, and O+MOP group maxilla received three MOPs placed 5 mm mesial to the first molar in addition to the force. (**a**) Reverse transcription polymerase chain reaction analysis of cytokine gene expression. Data is presented as fold increase in cytokine expression in the O and MOP groups in comparison to C group. Data shown is mean±SEM of three experiments. (**b**) Number of tartrate-resistant acid phosphatase-positive osteoclasts in the C, O, and O+MOP groups, identified as brown cells in immunohistochemical stained sections. Each value represents the mean±SEM of five animals (* significantly different from C group, ** significantly different from O group). (**c**) Axial views of right maxilla of control and different experimental groups were obtained by micro-CT. Note the significant increase in osteoporosity in the presence of MOPs. (**d**) Intraoral photographs show the increase magnitude of tooth movement in the O+MOP group in comparison to the O group

significant impact. Similarly, a human clinical trial using a canine retraction model demonstrates that MOPs can amplify the catabolic response to orthodontic forces. Canine retraction in the presence of MOPs results in twice as much distalization compared with patients receiving similar orthodontic forces without MOPs. This increase in tooth movement is accompanied by an increase in the level of inflammatory mediators [4].

Clinical studies demonstrate that increasing the number of MOPs significantly increases expression of inflammatory mediators and the magnitude of tooth movement (*Seminars in Orthodontics*, [3] http://dx.doi.org/10.1053/j.sodo.2015.06.002). Therefore, one should expect procedures such as orthognathic surgery, corticotomies, or piezocision to significantly increase the levels of inflammatory cytokines beyond those induced by MOPs. While increase in cytokine release by these methods is accompanied with higher rate of tooth movement, unfortunately, the increase in the expression of inflammatory mediators is not sustained for a long time. A significant decrease in cytokine activity is observed 2–3 months after any of these treatments. As a result, each of these procedures would need to be repeated during the course of orthodontic treatment, which renders some of the abovementioned modalities impractical.

3.4 Anabolic Phase of Orthodontic Tooth Movement

3.4.1 Osteoblast Activation

The catabolic phase of tooth movement that we just discussed is followed by an anabolic phase that allows the bone to keep its new morphological relation with adjacent structures. Importantly, the anabolic phase must involve both the trabecular and cortical bones. However, the molecular events that initiate the anabolic phase are not clear.

Alveolar bone in the area opposite to the direction of tooth movement is exposed to tensile stresses. Similar to activation of osteoclasts in compression side, the activation of osteoblasts in the tension side cannot be denied. But why are osteoblasts activated in the tension side? Some have suggested that osteoblast activation in these areas is simply a response to tensile stresses. However, many observations discredit this view. While some in vitro experiments demonstrate osteoblasts activation in response to tensile forces [17], these experiments have not been supported by in vivo studies. Experiments in long bones and alveolar bone demonstrate that at physiologic levels, osteocyte activation requires intermittent loads of specific frequency and acceleration [4, 14, 37]. Therefore, application of static tensile forces such as orthodontic forces would not be able to explain bone formation in the tension side. Furthermore, it has been shown that static tensile forces in long bones can cause bone resorption and not formation [7], while under high frequency and acceleration, tensile forces similar to compression forces can be osteogenic [16, 35]. Thus, other factors should explain the anabolic phase of orthodontic tooth movement. The *Biphasic Theory of Tooth Movement* was developed to address these inconsistencies.

3.5 *Biphasic Theory of Tooth Movement*

As we have just detailed, the biological phenomenon of tooth movement results from tightly coupled and choreographed response of osteocytes, osteoclasts, and osteoblasts to orthodontic forces. Specifically, the evidence points to the conversion of orthodontic forces into temporally sequenced biological phases of catabolism followed by anabolism in alveolar bone. Taken together, the data on tooth movement led us to developed the *Biphasic Theory of Tooth Movement* to not only more fully explain the biological consequences of orthodontic treatment but to also guide researchers to develop accelerated, efficacious, and safe orthodontic treatments.

3.5.1 Biology of Tooth Movement: Rethinking the Existing Data

The classic theory of biology of tooth movement has three main pillars (1) osteoclastogenesis occurs due to compression stresses and osteoblast activity occurs due to tensile stresses, and therefore osteoclasts should populate compression sites and osteoblasts should populate tension sites; (2) the catabolic phase and anabolic phase occur independently of each other in the PDL on opposite sides of the tooth; and (3) although independent, the catabolic and anabolic phases occur simultaneously, since both compression and tensile stresses occur simultaneously.

While these principles are still the foundation of current thinking, they are only partially true. Histologic sections at early time points of force application demonstrate activation of osteoclasts in both compression and tension sites, which suggests that both compression and tensile forces can traumatize the PDL (Fig. 3.4a). It also demonstrates unequivocally that osteoclastogenesis is not limited to the compression side. This can clearly be observed in uCT scans of the alveolar bone around moving teeth, which demonstrate increase in radiolucency all around the tooth and not only in the compression site (Fig. 3.4b).

It is also illogical to assume a strict geographical distribution of bone resorption and formation based on compression and tension. If tension produced only bone formation without any resorption, then the trailing, tension-bearing alveolar bone would become measurably (in fact, ridiculously) thicker following tooth movement. Likewise, if compression only produced bone resorption, then there would be complete resorption of alveolar bone at the leading compression-bearing region of the socket. In fact, neither of these occur, which means that both catabolic and anabolic responses occur in the alveolus around the entire tooth – regardless of the type of force that is actually experienced at a specific site – ensuring that the alveolus remains intact throughout orthodontic treatment.

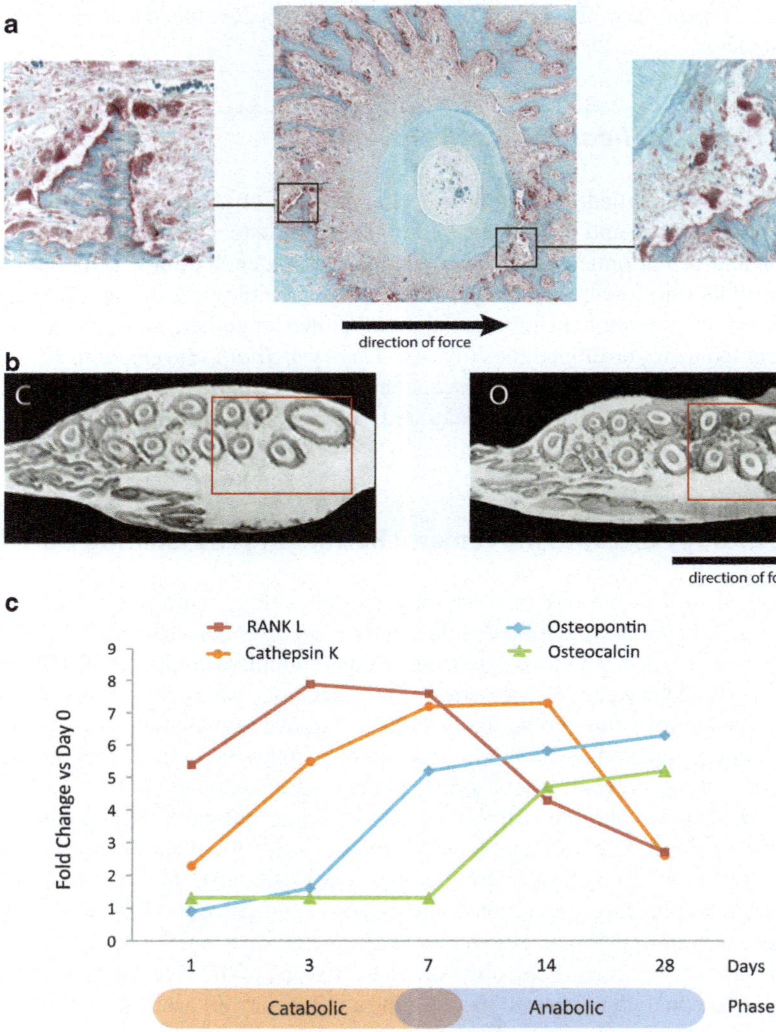

Fig. 3.4 Evidence supports the *Biphasic Theory of Tooth Movement*. Rat hemimaxillae were collected at different time points after application of force (25 cN) to mesialize the first molar. Control animals did not receive any force. (**a**) Immunohistochemical staining for tartrate-resistant acid phosphatase 3 days after force application. Axial section shows osteoclasts identified positive red cells in both the tension and compression side of the moving root. (**b**) Micro-CT images of right maxillary molars of control (*C*) and orthodontic force (*O*) animals, 14 days after application of force, show significant osteopenia surrounding the moving first molar (*red rectangular* are). (**c–e**) Reverse transcription polymerase chain reaction analysis of osteoclast (RANK L and cathepsin K) and osteoblast (osteocalcin and osteopontin) markers in the hemimaxillae of rats at different time points after force activation. Data is presented as fold increase in expression in response to orthodontic force compared to day 0 and as mean±SEM of three experiments. (**c**) The onset of significant differences in RANK L and cathepsin K were observed at day 3, and for osteopontin and osteocalcin at day 7 and day 14, respectively, supporting a catabolic phase preceding and anabolic phase during tooth movement. (**d, e**) Reverse transcription polymerase chain reaction analysis of rat maxillae where molars were moved in the absence (ortho) or presence (ortho+AI) of anti-inflammatory drugs, added to the drinking water (* significantly different from ortho group)

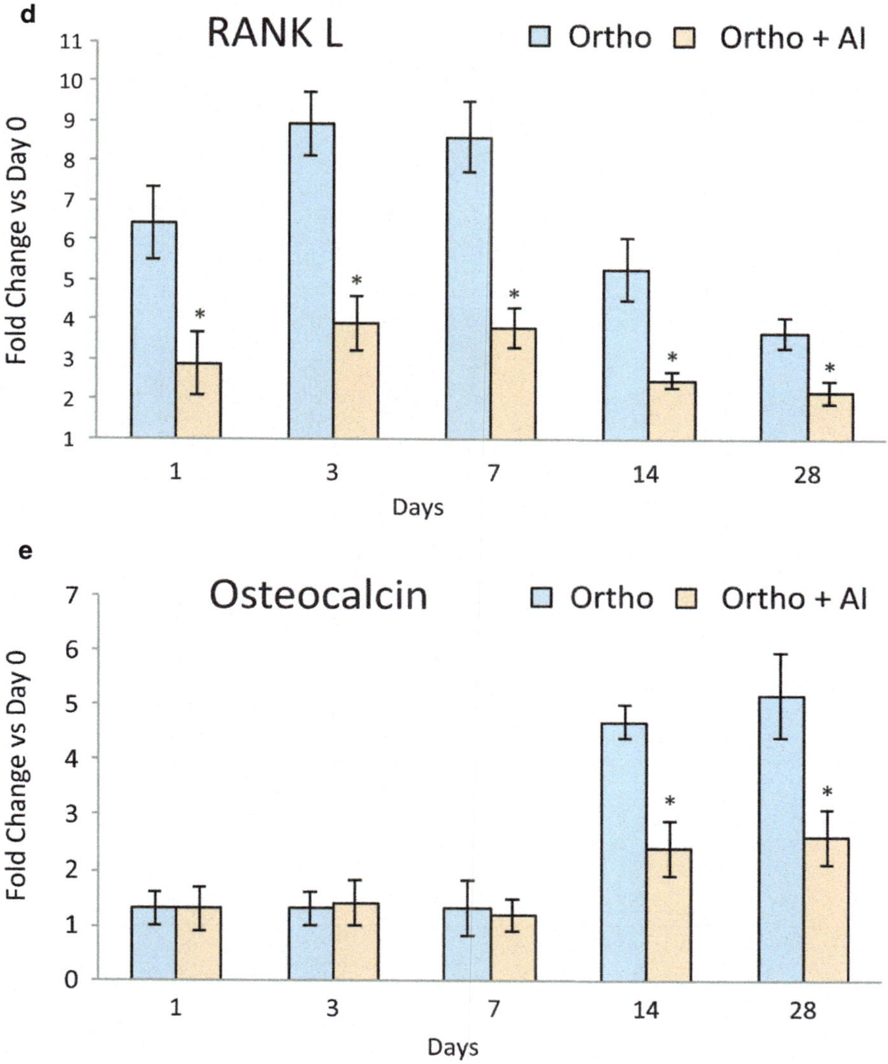

Fig. 3.4 (continued)

While both the catabolic and anabolic phases occur at all points around the tooth, they do not occur simultaneously. There is a measurable delay in the anabolic phase following the catabolic phase, as demonstrated by the high expression of osteoclast markers at early stage of tooth movement and high expression of osteogenic markers toward later stages of tooth movement (Fig. 3.4c). If the anabolic phase results directly from tensile stress, then one would expect osteoblast activation and the expression of bone formation and resorption markers to occur simultaneously, without any delay.

Furthermore, when anti-inflammatory medication is given (with a subsequent decrease in osteoclastogenesis), osteogenic activity decreases significantly as measured by decreased osteogenic marker expression (Fig. 3.4d, e)

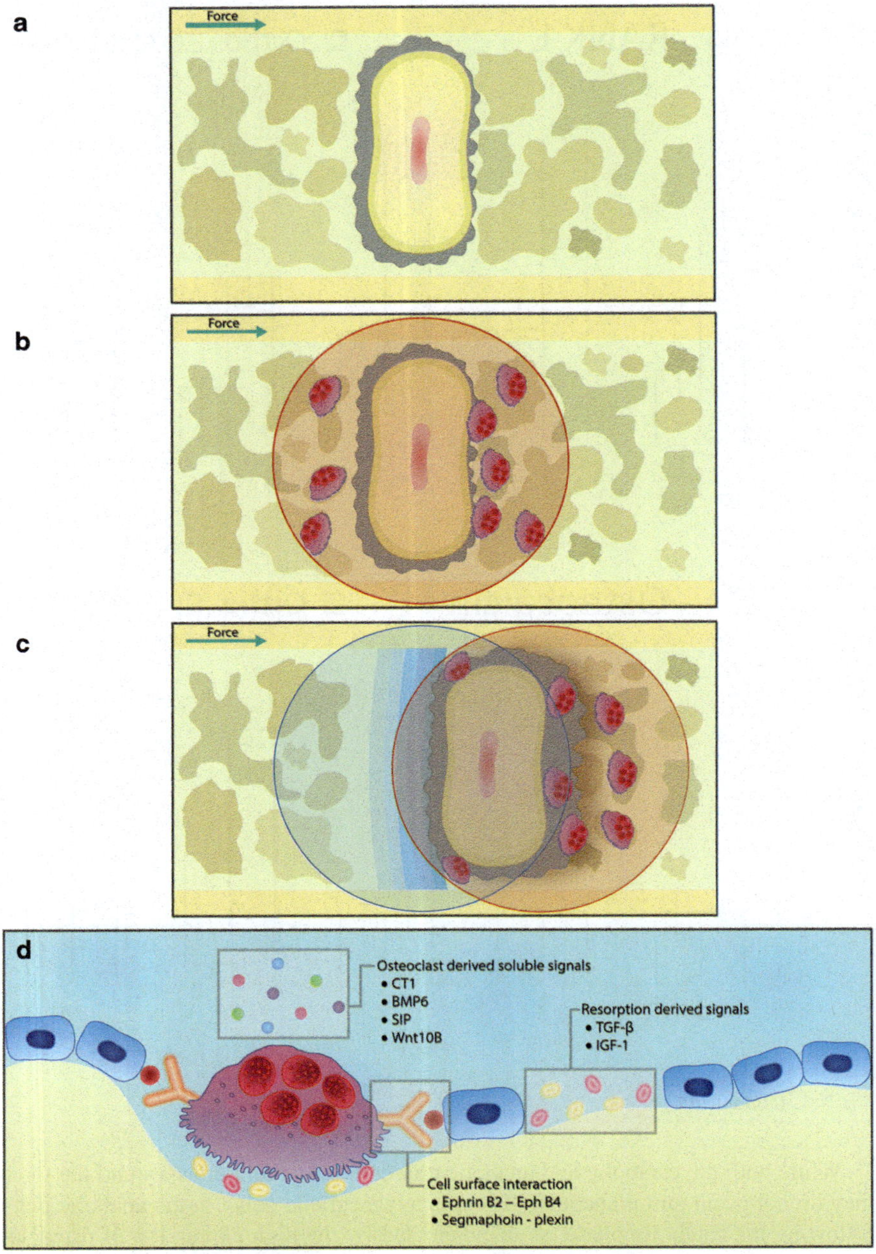
a
Force
b
Force
c
Force
d
Osteoclast derived soluble signals
• CT1
• BMP6
• SIP
• Wnt10B
Resorption derived signals
• TGF-β
• IGF-1
Cell surface interaction
• Ephrin B2 – Eph B4
• Segmaphoin - plexin

Based on these observations, it is logical to assume that the biologic response during tooth movement comprises two clearly separated phases that are not site specific. In other words, both compression and tensile stresses cause damage to the PDL, which stimulates a perimeter of osteoclastogenesis (Fig. 3.5b). The tooth will move in the direction of the orthodontic force into the space created by osteoclast activity, and with that movement, the perimeter of osteoclastogenesis drifts in the direction of the force. This phase is followed by an anabolic phase, where osteoblasts are activated to replace the destroyed bone, creating a perimeter of osteogenesis (Fig. 3.5c). The osteoclastogenesis perimeter is a prerequisite for the activation of the osteogenic perimeter. It is important to note that in considering our proposal that there is a strict temporal relationship between the osteoclastogenesis and osteogenic phases, histological sections would appear to contradict our conclusion by demonstrating that the two phases are independent events. Remember, histological sections are deceiving because they are static representations of a dynamic phenomenon. The data on osteoclast and osteogenic markers clearly support the temporal relationship that we propose (Fig. 3.4).

In the *Biphasic Theory of Tooth Movement*, osteoclasts play an important role in the activation of osteoblasts. This is in agreement with numerous studies that suggest osteoclasts are principle regulator of osteoblast activity [25]. In healthy individuals, osteoclast activation is tightly coupled to osteoblast activation. This effect can occur through different pathways: (1) osteoclasts release paracrine factors that directly recruit and activate osteoblasts, (2) osteoclasts activate osteoblasts through direct cell-cell interaction, and (3) bone resorption by osteoclasts exposes bone matrix proteins that then attract and activate osteoblasts (Fig. 3.5d). While these pathways differ fundamentally, they do share an important feature. In each case, osteoclast activity precedes osteoblast activity. This directionality is seen any time osteoclasts are activated and is best visualized in the remodeling cone where the

Fig. 3.5 *Biphasic Theory of Tooth Movement* explained by the coupling of osteoclast activity with osteoblast activity. The biologic response during tooth movement comprises two clearly separated phases. After application of an orthodontic force (**a**), both the compression and tensile stresses generated by displacement of the tooth cause damage to PDL stimulating a perimeter of osteoclastogenesis (*red circle*) (**b**). Once the tooth moves in the direction of the orthodontic force into the space created by osteoclast activity, a perimeter of osteogenesis and bone formation (*blue circle*) is created roughly in the same area of the alveolar bone where the catabolic response took place (**c**). The coupling of the catabolic response (osteoclast activity) with the anabolic response (osteoblast activity) during orthodontic tooth movement can occur through different pathways: osteoclast-derived signals working a paracrine fashion, direct cell-cell interaction, and growth factor release from the matrix during bone resorption (**d**)

head of the cone is occupied by osteoclasts and the tail of the cone is filled with osteoblasts. By harnessing this repeatable and predictable sequential process, we can increase the anabolic effect of orthodontics in both trabecular and cortical bones.

3.5.2 Enhancing the Anabolic Effect of Orthodontic Treatment

Enhancing the catabolic effect of orthodontic tooth movement is the basis for accelerating tooth movement using MOPs. To ensure dental and skeletal health at the end of MOPs and orthodontic treatment, as well as to ensure long-term occlusal stability, the anabolic effect of treatment must also be enhanced.

Stimulating the anabolic effect in trabecular bone allows us to move a tooth into an area of alveolar bone loss, as commonly seen at post-extraction sites. Likewise, enhancing the anabolic effect in cortical bone can increase the boundaries of orthodontic tooth movement. A more detailed look at the coupling of the catabolic and anabolic responses uncovers exciting possibilities for new orthodontic treatment methods.

3.5.3 MOP-Enhanced Anabolic Response

Activation of osteoblasts by osteoclasts is observed during tooth movement where the bone resorption phase of tooth movement is followed by a bone formation phase to prevent bone loss during tooth movement. Similar phenomenon can be stimulated during movement of a tooth into an area of alveolar bone loss. These areas usually are occupied with thick cortical bone that is short in height and narrow in width. Moving a tooth in this area is slow, can cause root resorption, and usually results in tilting the crown into the edentulous space without significant root movement. Applying MOPs in this edentulous area harnesses the catabolic phase of orthodontic treatment to decrease the bone density. This allows faster tooth movement into the area with less possibility of root resorption and greater bodily movement rather than tipping. This osteoclast activity then increases osteoblast activity significantly, which couples catabolism-dependent tooth movement with anabolism-dependent remodeling that restores the bone height and width in the previously edentulous site.

3.5.4 MOP-Generated Cortical Drift

Alveolar cortical bone sets the physical and physiologic limits of orthodontic tooth movement. While a tooth can be driven through the cortical plate if the orthodontic force applied to it has sufficient magnitude, direction, and duration, the speed of cortical bone remodeling is slow enough that appropriately directed forces rarely place any tooth in danger of breaching the physical limit set by the cortical bone. However, orthodontists face a conundrum when they have a borderline extraction case where expansion would provide the ideal space needed to unravel the crowding but the alveolar boundary conditions are not robust enough to tolerate the expansion. Therefore, it would be of great value for orthodontists to manipulate these boundary conditions by increasing bone formation at the surface of the cortical bone. Application of MOPs in the direction of orthodontic tooth movement can stimulate osteoclasts that will first decrease the bone density of cortical bone and second stimulate osteoblast activity in the direction of movement. This treatment results in the drift of the cortical plate into a new position with significant bone formation in the direction of tooth movement. This is especially important when moving teeth toward the cortical boundaries, for example, during expansion in adults or retraction of lower anterior teeth during correction of severe class III patients.

3.6 Summary

In this chapter, we reviewed current views on the biology of tooth movement, discussed scientific evidence that questions the validity of current theories, and presented a new theory on the biology of tooth movement – the *Biphasic Theory of Tooth Movement*. Based on this theory, the catabolic and anabolic phases of tooth movement are not limited to a particular area or to the type of stress generated as previously proposed. In addition, the catabolic phase always precedes the anabolic phase and is necessary for anabolic phase to occur.

Since both catabolic and anabolic phases can be manipulated by procedures such as MOPs, it is possible not only to increase the rate of tooth movement but also to expand the boundaries of tooth movement by stimulating bone formation in trabecular and cortical bone and introducing a new era of orthodontics where nonsurgical correction of severe skeletal deformities in a short period of time will become routine.

References

1. Alikhani M, Alansari S, Sangsuwon C, Bin Lee Y, Alikhani M, Khoo E, Teixeira C. Biological mechanisms to accelerate tooth movement. In: Stem cell biology and tissue engineering. Elsevier. 2015. p. 787–98.
2. Alikhani M, Alyami B, Lee IS, Almoammar S, Vongthongleur T, Alikhani M, Alansari S, Sangsuawon C, Chou M, Khoo E, Boskey A, Teixeia C. Biological saturation point during orthodontic tooth movement. Orthod Craniofac Res. 2015;18(1):8–17.
3. Alikhani M, Alansari S, Sangsuwon C, Alikhani M, Chou MY, Alyami B, Nervina JM, Teixeira CC. Micro-osteoperforations: minimally invasive accelerated tooth movement. Semin Orthod. 2015;21(3):162–9.
4. Alikhani M, Khoo E, Alyami B, Raptis M, Salgueiro JM, Oliveira SM, Boskey A, Teixeira CC. Osteogenic effect of high-frequency acceleration on alveolar bone. J Dent Res. 2012;91(4):413–9.
5. Alikhani M, Raptis M, Zoldan B, Sangsuwon C, Lee YB, Alyami B, Corpodian C, Barrera LM, Alansari S, Khoo E, Teixeira C. Effect of micro-osteoperforations. Authors' response. Am J Orthod Dentofacial Orthop. 2014;145(3):273–4.
6. Andrade Jr I, Silva TA, Silva GA, Teixeira AL, Teixeira MM. The role of tumor necrosis factor receptor type 1 in orthodontic tooth movement. J Dent Res. 2007;86(11):1089–94.
7. Andrade Jr I, Taddei SRA, Garlet GP, Garlet TP, Teixeira AL, Silva TA, Teixeira MM. CCR5 down-regulates osteoclast function in orthodontic tooth movement. J Dent Res. 2009;88(11):1037–41.

8. Bassett CA. Biologic significance of piezoelectricity. Calcif Tissue Res. 1968;1(4):252–72.
9. Chumbley AB, Tuncay OC. The effect of indomethacin (an aspirin-like drug) on the rate of orthodontic tooth movement. Am J Orthod. 1986;89(4):312–4.
10. De Albuquerque Taddei SR, Queiroz-Junior CM, Moura AP, Andrade Jr I, Garlet GP, Proudfoot AE, Teixeira MM, Da Silva TA. The effect of CCL3 and CCR1 in bone remodeling induced by mechanical loading during orthodontic tooth movement in mice. Bone. 2013;52(1):259–67.
11. Delaurier A, Allen S, Deflandre C, Horton MA, Price JS. Cytokine expression in feline osteoclastic resorptive lesions. J Comp Pathol. 2002;127(2–3):169–77.
12. Dubois RN, Abramson SB, Crofford L, Gupta RA, Simon LS, Van De Putte LBA, Lipsky PE. Cyclooxygenase in biology and disease. Faseb J. 1998;12(12):1063–73.
13. Fuller K, Kirstein B, Chambers TJ. Murine osteoclast formation and function: differential regulation by humoral agents. Endocrinology. 2006;147(4):1979–85.
14. Garlet TP, Coelho U, Silva JS, Garlet GP. Cytokine expression pattern in compression and tension sides of the periodontal ligament during orthodontic tooth movement in humans. Eur J Oral Sci. 2007;115(5):355–62.
15. Garman R, Rubin C, Judex S. Small oscillatory accelerations, independent of matrix deformations, increase osteoblast activity and enhance bone morphology. PLoS One. 2007;2(7), e653.
16. Gurton AU, Akin E, Sagdic D, Olmez H. Effects of PGI2 and TxA2 analogs and inhibitors in orthodontic tooth movement. Angle Orthod. 2004;74(4):526–32.
17. Hert J, Liskova M, Landrgot B. Influence of the long-term, continuous bending on the bone. An experimental study on the tibia of the rabbit. Folia Morphol (Praha). 1969;17(4):389–99.
18. Ikegame M, Ishibashi O, Yoshizawa T, Shimomura J, Komori T, Ozawa H, Kawashima H. Tensile stress induces bone morphogenetic protein 4 in preosteoblastic and fibroblastic cells, which later differentiate into osteoblasts leading to osteogenesis in the mouse calvariae in organ culture. J Bone Miner Res. 2001;16(1):24–32.
19. Iwasaki LR, Haack JE, Nickel JC, Reinhardt RA, Petro TM. Human interleukin-1 beta and interleukin-1 receptor antagonist secretion and velocity of tooth movement. Arch Oral Biol. 2001;46(2):185–9.
20. Jager A, Zhang D, Kawarizadeh A, Tolba R, Braumann B, Lossdorfer S, Gotz W. Soluble cytokine receptor treatment in experimental orthodontic tooth movement in the rat. Eur J Orthod. 2005;27(1):1–11.
21. Jimi E, Ikebe T, Takahashi N, Hirata M, Suda T, Koga T. Interleukin-1 alpha activates an NF-kappaB-like factor in osteoclast-like cells. J Biol Chem. 1996;271(9):4605–8.
22. Kale S, Kocadereli I, Atilla P, Asan E. Comparison of the effects of 1,25 dihydroxycholecalciferol and prostaglandin E2 on orthodontic tooth movement. Am J Orthod Dentofacial Orthop. 2004;125(5):607–14.
23. Kesavalu L, Chandrasekar B, Ebersole JL. In vivo induction of proinflammatory cytokines in mouse tissue by Porphyromonas gingivalis and Actinobacillus actinomycetemcomitans. Oral Microbiol Immunol. 2002;17(3):177–80.
24. Knop LA, Shintcovsk RL, Retamoso LB, Ribeiro JS, Tanaka OM. Non-steroidal and steroidal anti-inflammatory use in the context of orthodontic movement. Eur J Orthod. 2012;34(5):531–5.
25. Lundy FT, Linden GJ. Neuropeptides and neurogenic mechanisms in oral And periodontal inflammation. Crit Rev Oral Biol Med. 2004;15(2):82–98.
26. Matsuo K, Irie N. Osteoclast-osteoblast communication. Arch Biochem Biophys. 2008;473(2):201–9.
27. Mohammed AH, Tatakis DN, Dziak R. Leukotrienes in orthodontic tooth movement. Am J Orthod Dentofacial Orthop. 1989;95(3):231–7.
28. Mosley JR, March BM, Lynch J, Lanyon LE. Strain magnitude related changes in whole bone architecture in growing rats. Bone. 1997;20(3):191–8.
29. O'Brien CA, Gubrij I, Lin SC, Saylors RL, Manolagas SC. STAT3 activation in stromal/osteoblastic cells is required for induction of the receptor activator of NF-kappaB ligand and stimulation of osteoclastogenesis by gp130-utilizing cytokines or interleukin-1 but not 1,25-dihydroxyvitamin D3 or parathyroid hormone. J Biol Chem. 1999;274(27):19301–8.

30. O'Connor JA, Lanyon LE, Macfie H. The influence of strain rate on adaptive bone remodelling. J Biomech. 1982;15(10):767–81.
31. Perkins DJ, Kniss DA. Tumor necrosis factor-alpha promotes sustained cyclooxygenase-2 expression: attenuation by dexamethasone and NSAIDs. Prostaglandins. 1997;54(4):727–43.
32. Qin YX, Kaplan T, Saldanha A, Rubin C. Fluid pressure gradients, arising from oscillations in intramedullary pressure, is correlated with the formation of bone and inhibition of intracortical porosity. J Biomech. 2003;36(10):1427–37.
33. Quinn RS, Yoshikawa DK. A reassessment of force magnitude in orthodontics. Am J Orthod. 1985;88(3):252–60.
34. Ren Y, Maltha JC, Van'T Hof MA, Kuijpers-Jagtman AM. Optimum force magnitude for orthodontic tooth movement: a mathematic model. Am J Orthod Dentofacial Orthop. 2004;125(1):71–7.
35. Ricciotti E, Fitzgerald GA. Prostaglandins and inflammation. Arterioscler Thromb Vasc Biol. 2011;31(5):986–1000.
36. Rubin CT, Lanyon LE. Regulation of bone formation by applied dynamic loads. J Bone Joint Surg Am. 1984;66(3):397–402.
37. Rubin CT, Lanyon LE. Kappa Delta Award paper. Osteoregulatory nature of mechanical stimuli: function as a determinant for adaptive remodeling in bone. J Orthop Res: Off Publ Orthop Res Soc. 1987;5(2):300–10.
38. Rubin C, Turner AS, Bain S, Mallinckrodt C, Mcleod K. Anabolism. Low mechanical signals strengthen long bones. Nature. 2001;412(6847):603–4.
39. Sekhavat AR, Mousavizadeh K, Pakshir HR, Aslani FS. Effect of misoprostol, a prostaglandin E1 analog, on orthodontic tooth movement in rats. Am J Orthod Dentofacial Orthop. 2002;122(5):542–7.
40. Suzawa T, Miyaura C, Inada M, Maruyama T, Sugimoto Y, Ushikubi F, Ichikawa A, Narumiya S, Suda T. The role of prostaglandin E receptor subtypes (EP1, EP2, EP3, and EP4) in bone resorption: an analysis using specific agonists for the respective EPs. Endocrinology. 2000;141(4):1554–9.
41. Taddei SR, Andrade Jr I, Queiroz-Junior CM, Garlet TP, Garlet GP, Cunha Fde Q, Teixeira MM, Da Silva TA. Role of CCR2 in orthodontic tooth movement. Am J Orthod Dentofacial Orthop. 2012;141(2):153–60.
42. Teixeira CC, Khoo E, Tran J, Chartres I, Liu Y, Thant LM, Khabensky I, Gart LP, Cisneros G, Alikhani M. Cytokine expression and accelerated tooth movement. J Dent Res. 2010;89(10):1135–41.
43. Verna C, Dalstra M, Lee TC, Melsen B. Microdamage in porcine alveolar bone due to functional and orthodontic loading. Eur J Morphol. 2005;42(1–2):3–11.
44. Yasuda H, Shima N, Nakagawa N, Yamaguchi K, Kinosaki M, Mochizuki S, Tomoyasu A, Yano K, Goto M, Murakami A, Tsuda E, Morinaga T, Higashio K, Udagawa N, Takahashi N, Suda T. Osteoclast differentiation factor is a ligand for osteoprotegerin/osteoclastogenesis-inhibitory factor and is identical to TRANCE/RANKL. Proc Natl Acad Sci U S A. 1998;95(7):3597–602.
45. Yee JA, Turk T, Elekdag-Turk S, Cheng LL, Darendeliler MA. Rate of tooth movement under heavy and light continuous orthodontic forces. Am J Orthod Dentofacial Orthop. 2009;136(2):e151–9; discussion 150–1.
46. Yoshimatsu M, Shibata Y, Kitaura H, Chang X, Moriish T, Hashimoto F, Yoshida N, Yamaguchi A. Experimental model of tooth movement by orthodontic forces in mice and its application in tumor necrosis factor-deficient mice. J Bone Miner Metab. 2006;24(1):20–7.

Orthodontitis: The Inflammation Behind Tooth Movement and Orthodontic Root Resorption

4

Naphtali Brezniak and Atalia Wasserstein

Abstract

This chapter summarizes, criticizes, and updates the knowledge regarding orthodontitis – the inflammation that lies behind orthodontic tooth movement and orthodontic root resorption, gathered over the years, focusing on the last decade publications that followed the ending of the Human Genome Project. Types of root resorption as well as the remodeling and (mini)modeling processes involved in the orthodontic root resorption process are described. Several well-known theories that might explain root shortening as a result of orthodontic treatment are presented. The effects of patient-related factors and treatment-related factors (orthodontic and non-orthodontic) are discussed in light of current literature. A protocol to minimize orthodontic root resorption and to avoid consequences of periodontitis during orthodontic treatment, using radiographic monitoring (standard, frequent, or intensive), is suggested.

Inflammation is the process that lies behind orthodontic tooth movement [1–5]. Further, no orthodontic tooth movement is possible without this inflammation [6, 7]. Orthodontic force application, most of the time, reduces blood flow for enough time to induce local changes in the periodontal ligament (PDL) [8]. The body reaction to this process is usually by aseptic local inflammation. Until recently, when "orthodontitis" [9] was presented to the profession, this inflammation which lies behind tooth

N. Brezniak, MD, DMD, MSD (✉)
In Private Practice in Tel-Aviv, Tel-Aviv, Israel
e-mail: brezniak@gmail.com

A. Wasserstein, DMD
Orthodontic Departments, Hebrew and Tel-Aviv Universities, Tel-Aviv, Jerusalem, Israel
e-mail: ataliawa@gmail.com

B. Shroff (ed.), *Biology of Orthodontic Tooth Movement*,
DOI 10.1007/978-3-319-26609-1_4

movement and orthodontic root resorption (ORR) induced by orthodontic treatment was never named.

Orthodontitis, composed from the prefix which is our profession and the suffix "-itis" [10] that is used in medical terminology to describe any inflammation of an organ or a tissue. Since this inflammation involves the bone, the periodontal ligament and the tooth, the best name to fully describe the process is probably "orthodontitis."

According to histological observations, most studies demonstrate root surface changes cemental and dentinal in all teeth that are exposed to any level of force application [11, 12]. Although the effect of orthodontitis on the alveolar bone is different on the pressure and the tension sides, the effect on roots' surfaces is similar, but not equal, on both sides. Usually, more remodeling/modeling activity is detected on the pressure than on the tension sides.

From radiographic or clinical point of view, the manifestation of orthodontitis on the roots can be divided into two groups:

(a) Instrumental orthodontitis (IO) – where no radiographic signs on the roots' surfaces are evident
(b) Instrumental-detrimental orthodontitis (IDO) – where radiographic signs on the roots' surfaces are evident

Instrumental Orthodontitis (IO): IO initiates controlled bone modeling (resorption and apposition) [13], as well as bone and cemental remodeling (reversible changes) [13, 14]. IO enables tooth movement to occur due to frontal and undermining alveolar bone resorption as well as bone apposition on the pressure and the tension sides, respectively [15]. The roots next to IO areas also undergo surface resorption and apposition [16] mainly by cemental remodeling. These biological processes terminate when orthodontic force application ceases. The periodontal ligament that surrounds the roots, in most cases, is fully regenerated. IO symptoms include mild to moderate tooth mobility and/or sensitivity and pain during the first days following force application. The pain usually subsides in 1–3 days; however the mobility and some degree of sensitivity last during most time of the treatment [17]. IO clinical signs include mild to moderate tooth mobility [18] as the symptoms and minor to mild radiographic PDL (lamina dura) widening. No root shortening or other morphological changes can be detected radiographically. Signs and symptoms disappear following orthodontic force cessation. The mechanism behind the IO process is that the orthodontic force enables, in this case, almost normal blood flow but induces local electrical current and pH changes as well as release of different biological materials due to local environmental change (e.g., cytokines, prostaglandins, and others) [1, 2, 14]. These events trigger local inflammatory activity in the area surrounding the roots that are limited to the PDL, affecting the alveolar bone and cementum. The inflammation in the pressure area induces mainly bone modeling process, where the alveolar bone is resorbed, while the inflammation in the tension area induces bone modeling by the apposition process; new bone is deposited on the affected surfaces.

Surface cemental remodeling, similar to the physiological one, is induced in both areas as well. The inflammation mechanism, which is a part of a normal bone and cementum metabolism, is genetically controlled. It is activated regularly (not related to orthodontic treatment) during our lifetime and it remains behind the normal hard tissues remodeling/modeling process [13]. Regarding treatment, analgesics are sometimes prescribed during orthodontic treatment [19]. The patients/parents have to be aware of the pain, the sensitivity and the tooth mobility prior to force application, and the ability to use analgesics as well as soft diet during the period of pain and sensitivity. No further action is needed. If the pain, sensitivity, and/or tooth mobility lasts following treatment, the orthodontist should look for other reasons like dental trauma, periapical lesions, cervical resorption, or other tooth, periodontal, or endodontal pathologies.

IDO is divided into two:

1. Instrumental and Detrimental Orthodontitis Grade 1 (IDO1): The inflammation in IDO1, for yet unknown reasons, changes its character on the cemental side and the remodeling process changes its characteristics to the modeling process; the resorption process goes beyond the cementum into the dentin. It might be that during orthodontic force application, the local environmental changes, due to the decrease in the local blood supply and bone bending, induce the formation of large enough necrotic tissue. The necrotic tissue which has to be eliminated consequently releases different chemicals and biological components which encourage the inflammation activity by recruiting local and far away inflammatory cells. This time the inflammation process on the root surface goes beyond the expected and wanted remodeling into the modeling process. IDO1 produces minor to moderate root shortening [20] as well as scattered lacunae on other root surfaces. This irreversible ORR is the direct result of orthodontitis. ORR is usually diagnosed using X-rays during, close to the end, or following orthodontic treatment. The symptoms and treatment are similar to IO. When the orthodontic treatment is completed, there are only radiographic signs (root shortening or peripheral surface resorption) but no symptoms. Following treatment the patients/parents have to be informed about the morphological changes seen in the different X-rays films. No further treatment is needed. If IDO1 manifestations are diagnosed during treatment, one should follow the suggested protocol (Appendix).
2. Instrumental and Detrimental Orthodontitis Grade 2 (IDO2): IDO2 is very similar to IDO1. However, in this case, the inflammation results in severe root shortening [20]. The symptoms are tooth mobility and sensitivity during or following orthodontic treatment. The signs include tooth mobility/sensitivity and severe root shortening as viewed on X-rays. The consequences of IDO2 require treatment. The treatment for IDO2 depends on the time that it is discovered. If IDO2 is diagnosed during treatment, one should follow the suggested protocol (Appendix). However, if IDO2 is diagnosed after debonding, it is suggested that orthodontic or prosthodontic fixed retention be used to splint the affected teeth together with unaffected teeth. In rare situations, fused crowns can be a good

treatment solution. Extractions and implant replacements should be considered only in extremely rare cases if ever, since it has been demonstrated that those teeth can remain in the mouth for many years [21, 22]. The mechanism for both IDO1 and IDO2 is similar to that described for IO. However, due to personal susceptibilities, the level of the resorptive activity on the root surface is different, and it is probably individually genetically determined [23–26]. It is suggested that the physiological remodeling process, which has five steps, namely, activation, resorption, reversal, apposition, and quiescence, is being disturbed most likely in the transition between the resorption and the reversal stages [13, 14]. This coupling between resorption and apposition probably disappears or is delayed and, therefore, resorption continues into the next mineral tissue, the dentin, and it is characterized by irreversible morphological root changes that can be detected radiographically.

Background and terminology:

Historically, the phenomenon, we previously called orthodontically induced inflammatory root resorption (OIIRR), appeared as root absorption in the professional literature in the midst of the nineteenth century [27]; however, its significance began to receive clinical attention only in the beginning of and through the twentieth century [28, 29]. The knowledge related to OIIRR, since it was discovered, was expanded immensely, but yet, in spite of the scientific and the technological developments, most of the publications that try to uncover ways to prevent this phenomenon find difficulties in providing solutions. In almost all published data, there was a large variance between individuals in the study groups and in different teeth of the same individual. Even years after the Human Genome Project [30] ended, we do not know how to identify an individual patient with OIIRR potential or how to prevent the process.

The initial term "root absorption" [27] was replaced in the beginning of the twentieth century by the term root resorption (RR) [28]. Since then the process was defined as apical RR (ARR) [31], external ARR (EARR) [32], orthodontically induced RR (OIRR) [33], orthodontically induced inflammatory RR (OIIRR) [6, 7], and others. Only lately, the new name orthodontitis was presented to the profession [9]. This new term actually covers the depth and breadth of what lies behind the OIIRR phenomenon.

Although the clinical relevance of orthodontitis and its manifestations and ORR are controversial, the number of studies related to this topic has significantly increased. A review of all the articles is not realistic and there are many reviews on the subject with the most recent one published in 2010 [34]. This chapter will try to describe and discuss contemporary relevant materials and innovations that were published in the last decade and to focus on the analysis of this information.

Orthodontitis is affected by both patient- and treatment-related factors. The main *patient-related factors* published lately are associated with the followings: heredity [14, 23–25, 35–43], immunology [44–46], systemic factors [12, 47–64], chronologic age [65, 66], dental age [67, 68], gender [69, 70], presence of RR before orthodontic treatment [71, 72], habits [47, 73], previously traumatized teeth [74, 75], tooth structure/root form [70, 76–80], topography of adjacent alveolar bone [81–84], and individual tooth susceptibility [85–87]. The *treatment-related factors* should be divided into two groups: orthodontic treatment-related factors and non-orthodontic treatment-related factors. The orthodontic treatment-related factors published lately are associated with force magnitude [88–95], duration of force application [86, 88, 96–98], type of tooth movement [89, 99–101], and the treatment method [84, 86, 88, 102–118]. The non-orthodontic treatment-related factors published recently were endodontically treated teeth [42, 74, 75, 119, 120]; the use of nonsteroid anti-inflammatory drugs [50], doxycycline [51], and bisphosphonates [64]; surgical procedures (ovariectomy [62, 63], sympathectomy [121]); and the therapeutic effect of adding fluoride [58], thyroid hormone [60, 82], light-emitting diode (LED) [122], and ultrasound [123, 124] as a part of the treatment.

It is obvious that the periodical changes in the medical discourse have an important impact on the nature of the orthodontic studies and research. For example, when the influences of nutrition and metabolism on the human health were in the focus of the medical discourse, this same subject – the effect of nutrition and metabolism on orthodontitis and ORR – was studied in orthodontics as well [31, 125, 126]. When the medical literature was loaded with publications related to autoimmune diseases, the idea that there is the exposure of the dentin, tissue which is not recognized by the body's immune system, to humoral factors as an antigen appeared in the orthodontic literature as well [45].

And of course today, when the genes and associated subjects of the Human Genome Project like molecular biology and personalized medicine [127] are leading the medical discourse, we see that the number of studies relating to genetics is rapidly rising [14, 23, 25, 26, 35–41, 128, 129]. Maybe in the near future, as we see substantial amount of medical studies with good results on vaccines against factors involved in the inflammation process, like interleukins or cytokines [130], studies related to orthodontitis and ORR will be focused in that field.

The social hype and expectation raised by the Human Genome Project, initiated at the end of the last century, were enormous [131, 132], and they increased with the introduction of a private company – Celera – due to a competition with official government agencies that budget three billion USD to the project [133]. This project had short- and long-term goals [134]. Today, more than 10 years after the genome was decoded, it is clear that only a small part of the short-term goals, related primarily to mapping the human genome and to the innovative technology, have been fulfilled, while the major long-term goal is far from being achieved [30]. The ability to explain, using the knowledge obtained from the project, the differences in diversity of physiological and pathological processes between different individuals proved to be restricted [134]. Now, we further understand that the genes act in different ways in changing environment [135] (e.g., stress, fever, compression, and tension). The knowledge that no direct relationship between the genotype and the phenotype exists makes the discovery of individual characteristics challenging. The fact that each gene has a relationship in activity and expression to other nearby and even far away genes makes the statistical possible gene interactive relationships almost countless [136]. It is now clearer that genes are only actors, among many others that play on the human biology stage or network. The current discourse in technoscience-medical world [137] discusses not only the genome but also the proteome, a new and by far more complex world than that of the genome [138, 139]. Results of the studies show that the connection of genetics and orthodontitis can provide explanations in only small percentages of the phenomenon [23, 140, 141]. This is mainly due to the large variance between individuals and even between identical twins.

Along our life span, surface root remodeling is among many other physiological processes that take place in our body [13, 142]. This remodeling is seen in all teeth, erupted or not, that serve as control in orthodontitis studies [58, 143] and is a part of the normal human body physiological turnover. This remodeling is controlled by the inflammation mechanism, and when ended, the resorbed area is fully regenerated [13, 14]. It might be that this physiological turnover process is the result of direct (e.g., chewing) as well as indirect (mesial drift) pressure acting on the jaws that is transferred to the roots of the teeth. The only microscopic sign that indicates the existence of this resorption, apart from areas where it is directly observed, is the presence of a reversal line, a sedimentation of material generated by mononuclear lining cells from the blastic cells' lineage (fibroblast, osteoblast, cementoblats, etc.) at the very depth of the resorption area, where apposition of mineral material and the reconstruction of the resorbed area had begun [13]. The cementum covering the root is very similar to the alveolar bone structure [144], and both, like the cortical bone, experience the remodeling process which under normal circumstances is described as a coupling process that has its own precise sequence, from activation through resorption, reversal, formation, and its conclusion at the quiescence stage A-R-R-F-Q [13]. As mentioned, the process occurs at the roots of erupted teeth that are exposed to daily mechanical loads but also the roots of unerupted teeth that are exposed to indirect occlusal loads, as well as eruption forces. In most cases, this physiological resorption process takes place only at the cementum level and seldom reaches the defined boundaries of the dentin. This process is fully reversible and leaves no morphological scars that can be observed by external imaging methods. The process is a part of the normal cycle in both the apical cellular and the coronal acellular cemental layers.

Orthodontic force application changes, in minutes, the anatomical and physiological environment of the roots. All tissues involved in the system, namely, the roots, the periodontal ligament, and the bone (tooth, periodontal ligament, and bone system (TPLBS)), and sometimes areas that are far from this system, the sutures and other bones of the skull, experience those changes and react accordingly. This unexpected load stimulus that does not belong to the normal growth and development pathway demands the body to react. The reaction does not necessarily have to be in the limits of the physiological borders of the inflammation controlled remodeling process, where the TPLBS remains at the end of the process untouched, keeping the morphology and the function unchanged, as seen in most instances of force application (as described in IO). Actually in many cases, the reaction to orthodontic force application, the remodeling, goes far beyond the cementum into the dentin and actual loss of root material can be detected either microscopically or macroscopically. These morphological changes are irreversible and can be diagnosed, using several imaging techniques, especially cone bean computerized tomography, as shortening of the involved roots horizontally and/or rarely diagonally. Usually, the resorbed root material is replaced by alveolar bone; nevertheless, normal periodontal ligament layer always separates between the two, keeping the normal function of the harmed tooth [6, 7]. Actually, if we look at the different definitions related to bone turnover and other biological processes, the changes in the root can be associated with modulation or mini-modulation that initiated as remodeling reaction to the force application, and from a yet unknown reason, the coupling of reversal from resorption to formation did not occur. It is important to emphasize that teeth that experienced mild or even severe resorption do not lose their vitality, color, or function, similarly to the nearby periodontal ligament that moved in space [13]; furthermore, their roots' surface areas, in many instances, are relatively increased by the side surface local resorption, which might increase their stability as a compensation for shortening the roots.

Many publications are trying to explain the reasons or goals for *bone remodeling*. Is the goal of the process to repair micro-fractures in the bone due to fatigue, extreme loads, or local weakness, or is it a part of mineral, especially calcium, recruitment process, since the bone is the biggest mineral reservoir of the body? Or maybe is it a process that aims to remove osteocytes or cementocytes that went through apoptosis and ended their life cycle from the bone and cellular cemental areas, respectively?

We know that in extreme circumstances, the body sacrifices less essential tissues and organs [145]. When the TPLBS is exposed to an extreme condition, such as increased force application, the local strain increases above a certain amount for a long enough time (the threshold of the amount of force and time is individually determined). The first programmed reaction activates the physiological inflammation process. Local materials that are being released from the damaged cells initiate a process of recruiting local and far away cells in order to eliminate the and repair the initial damage. However, when the blood supply is decreased and the amount of the hyalinized necrotic tissue increases, there might be difficulties in maintaining the normal coupling process, even by accelerating it or by increasing the areas of the resorption on the cementum surface [94, 97]. Thus the remodeling process experiences insufficiency. The expression of this insufficiency, while still reversible, is detected first only by using the microscope and when it continues and the damage to the roots is large enough and goes beyond the cementum into the dentin. The initially reversible process turns into an irreversible one that can be detected even by using external imaging techniques. We do not know yet whether the reaction to the insufficiency remains within the boundaries of the known inflammation mechanism or activates a new, yet unknown, pre-programmed destructive reaction aimed to protect the surrounding alveolar bone and periodontal ligament by scarifying the roots. Further, we definitely should ask the questions: Why in most IDO1 and IDO2 cases the roots are being replaced by bone tissue and not, for example, by connective tissue? And moreover, how come the periodontal ligament and adjacent bone are fully regenerated while only the roots are being changed and resorbed? Are the bone and the periodontal tissue placed higher than the roots in the hierarchy of tissue importance (if it exists) (Fig. 4.1)?

Another theory can be suggested. This one is based on the well-known evolutional phenomenon called the Butler's field theory [146]. This theory tries to explain the reason for the disappearance of the last tooth in each field of the dentition (lateral incisors, second premolars, and third molars) during evolution [147]. It might be speculated that when the TPLBS is exposed to an extreme condition, in which the local blood supply stops and necrotic tissue appears, the body activates hidden genetic mechanisms which normally are used to decrease the number of teeth, however in this instance only partially.

The "self-defense mechanism" is another theological possibility that might explain this irreversible root shortening. It may well be that by activating the IDO1 and IDO2, the body intends to prevent itself from reoccurrence of similar events in the future. Since force application increases the inside pressure in the TPLBS, the body initially utilizes physical and later biological mechanisms in trying to do their best to reduce the entropy (the disorder) immediately, with implication to the future. It might be that by reducing the root length, the disrupting local pressure is decreased, and future similar threat is prevented. The publication that found less root shortening in patients with a history of earlier orthodontic treatment compared to the remaining patients [148] supports this theory. There were early reports that recognized the overall protective function of the root's outer layer, the cementoid, or the precementum [8], but there are no explanations why the roots are more protected in the second orthodontic round. According to our proposed theory, the root shortening by itself can prevent a future pressure around the apex from being raised. In Figs. 4.2 and 4.3, we can see the effect of root shortening on the amount

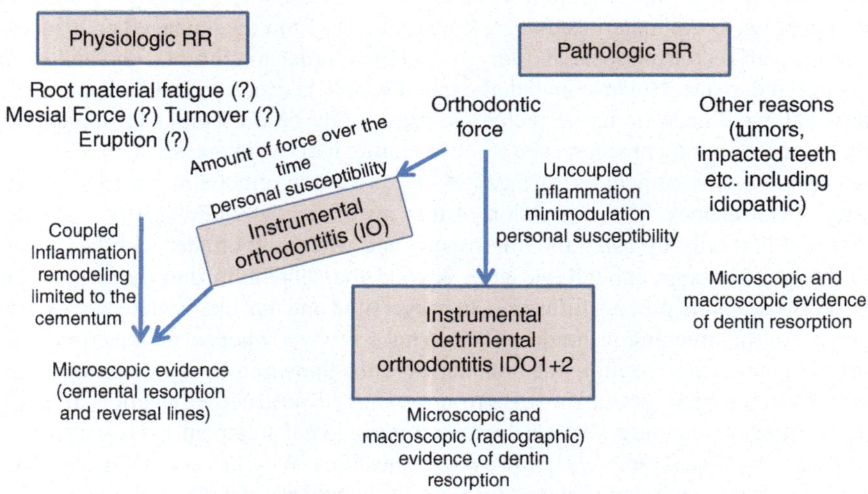

Fig. 4.1 Types of root resorption (RR)

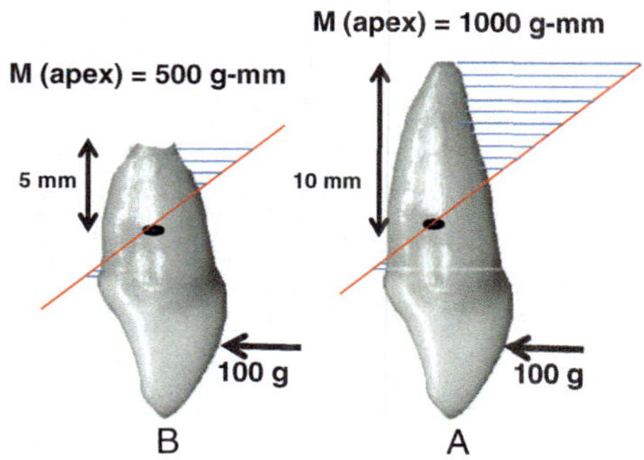

Fig. 4.2 Stress, force, and moments and the self-defense mechanism theory in uncontrolled force application. If an uncontrolled 100 g of force is applied to tooth A, the center of rotation is close to the center of resistance, and the stress distribution on the root surface is depicted by the horizontal lines. Note the minimal stress line next to both the center of rotation and the gingival area of the root. If the same force is applied to tooth B with a shorter resorbed root, the amount of stress developed in the apical area is much lower than that on tooth A with the longer root (see text)

of stress developed in the apical zone due to similar uncontrolled and torque force applications. Figures 4.2 and 4.3 graphics depict the issue [149]:

The strain and of course the stress developed in the TPLBS following orthodontic force application are dependent on mechanical factors like the amount of the force applied, point of application, the resultant vector of force and moment, the location of the center of resistance, and others, as well as biological factors, like the root shape and form, the number of roots, the biological and physical properties of the cementum, periodontal ligament and bone, and more. It is clear that mostly genetics determines the major biological factor, related to the potential reaction to the strain. It determines the degree of the inflammatory reaction and the degree of the resistance or

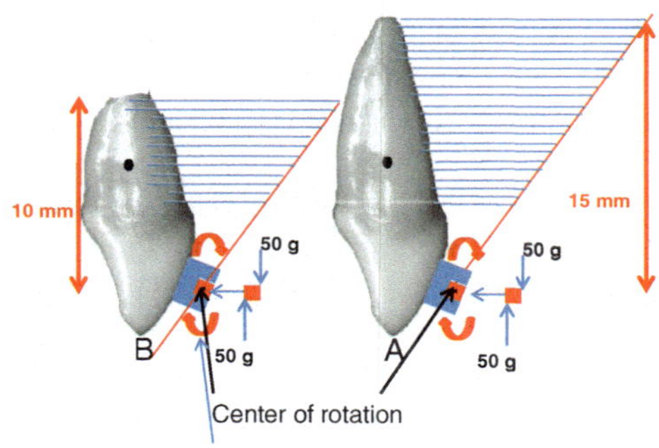

Fig. 4.3 Stress, force, and moments and the self-defense mechanism theory in torque application. In order to move the root of tooth A and tooth B bucally, torque is needed. The center of rotation in this movement is in the bracket, which is away from the center of resistance. Using similar forces on both teeth, the amount of developed stress in the apical zone of tooth A is much bigger than the one developed in the tooth with shorter root B (see text)

the vulnerability of the individual to orthodontitis. Genetics, epigenetics, and environmental factors determine the general health condition of the individual and his/her ability to react to the force. It is well known that even identical twins, whose genome is equal, react in different ways, due to environmental influences [150] and even hybrids mice do not always react exactly the same in identical conditions. Individual variances are always there. A major factor that should not be forgotten, associated to the reaction of the body to orthodontic force, is time. Roughly we can divide the population into three categories related to their susceptibility to orthodontitis:

(a) Those that are not susceptible at all and will never show any macroscopic signs (signs that can be detected by X-rays) during the whole treatment, whether light, medium, or heavy forces will be applied for short, medium, or long term. Those patients own a high threshold level to force over the time and will react always by developing only IO as a reaction to the applied forces.
(b) Those who will always show macroscopic signs of root shortening, in any orthodontic treatment, when light, medium, or heavy forces will be used for short, medium, or long term. Those patients own a low threshold level to force over the time and will develop manifestations of IDO1 and occasionally IDO2 as a reaction to the applied forces.
(c) Those whose genetic-environmental complex reaction or threshold is sensitive to the amount of force and/or duration of treatment time. For example, when using low levels of force for a short treatment time, both or the mutual combination of force and time is under the threshold of activating IDO (1 0R 2) (the actual amount of force level and time length are yet not known). This will prevent the appearance of macroscopic root shortening, however, if the force will be above their threshold or the time will be long enough or there will be a mutual combination, namely, low force but long treatment time or high force but a short treatment time; macroscopic root shortening as a result of IDO [1, 2] will be evident (see Fig. 4.4).

During our lifetime there might be shifting from one group to another. It depends on health condition, nutrition, metabolism, mental state, and of course other unknown yet genetic and/or environmental variables.

It is well known that all the abovementioned biological- and treatment-related factors change with time and actually all the time, even during the orthodontic treatment or experiments. Therefore, our abilities to in-depth study the subject are limited, and drawing conclusion from those studies should be taken with utmost care. Most of the clinical studies, dealing with orthodontitis, are retrospective, and therefore we can only compare the final state with the initial one or to a 6–9-month periapical X-ray of the upper incisors, suggested by Malmgren [20], if it was taken [151, 152]. We do not have the ability to follow or to know from those studies the exact time root changes had happened. Is it at the beginning, midterm, or final stages of the treatment? Was it a short-term event or did it last slowly through the whole treatment time? From Malmgren [20] publication, it is clear that the number of teeth suffers from IDO

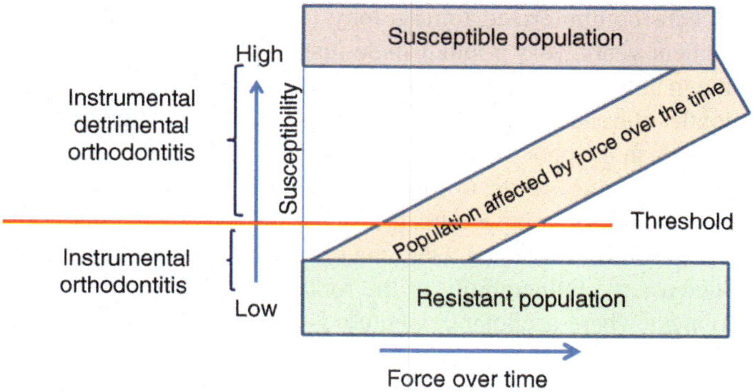

Fig. 4.4 Population susceptibility categories

increases with treatment time. We can speculate that during the last period of treatment, the ability to involve torque movements in the treatment is increased. Torque, unlike uncontrolled movements, moves the center of rotation, away from the center of resistance, toward the bracket and by that increases the distance from the apical region. The direct result of this movement, the torque, is the heavily increased moment developed in the apical region relative to an uncontrolled movement, which might affect the local stress and further the activation of the destructive consequence (Fig. 4.5).

We know the gender and age of the patients, the treatment durations, the appliances used, whether it was an extraction or non-extraction case, and some other general socioeconomic and demographic parameters. We know that in most cases when we detect, following treatment, root length changes, they always appear in the apical region. It can be either full root shortening or diagonal one that is diagnosed

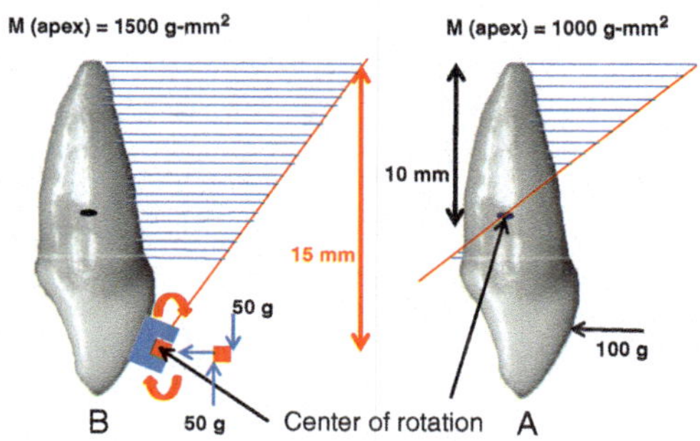

Fig. 4.5 The difference in stress distribution of uncontrolled force and torque on the apex. If an uncontrolled 100 g of force is applied to tooth A, the center of rotation is close to the center of resistance, and the stress distribution on the root surface is depicted by the horizontal lines. Note the minimal stress next to both the center of rotation and the gingival area of the root. In order to move the root of tooth B bucally, torque is needed. Since the center of rotation in this movement is in the bracket, which is away from the center of resistance, for the same force, the stress distribution on the root surface is much higher especially in the apical zone

using cone beam computerized tomography (CBCT) [153], an imaging tool that became, in recent years, very popular in dentistry.

How come in most short-term experimental in vivo clinical studies, following a few weeks or months of treatment [89, 95], morphological root changes can be detected in the extracted teeth in the pressure and tension surfaces surrounding the roots, but never as apical root shortening, while in long-term clinical studies in which teeth are not extracted, apical root shortening is detected following 6 and more months of treatment? This disparity was never explained. Does the presence of cellular cementum in the apical region increase the vulnerability of the roots to orthodontic forces in this region compared to areas where acellular cementum is present? Does the fact that the coronary areas of the root, surrounded with very thin alveolar bone, having the ability to bend and absorb part of the pressure developed due to the force applied to the teeth defend those areas of the roots from the damage of orthodontitis (IDO)? Does the fact that the coronal root area is open to the oral cavity, and the different fluids, i.e., extracellular, intracellular, and blood, can easily move outside the scene and by that decrease the pressure developed, compared to the apical areas, where the bone is much thicker and the area is almost blocked to fast fluid movement, from higher to lower pressure zones, explain why we see mainly apical root shortening compared to less coronal root damage, or is it due to the fact that the stress distribution levels in most movements are higher in the apical region compared to the coronal region if the pressure level is the main factor initiating the IDO process (Fig. 4.6)?

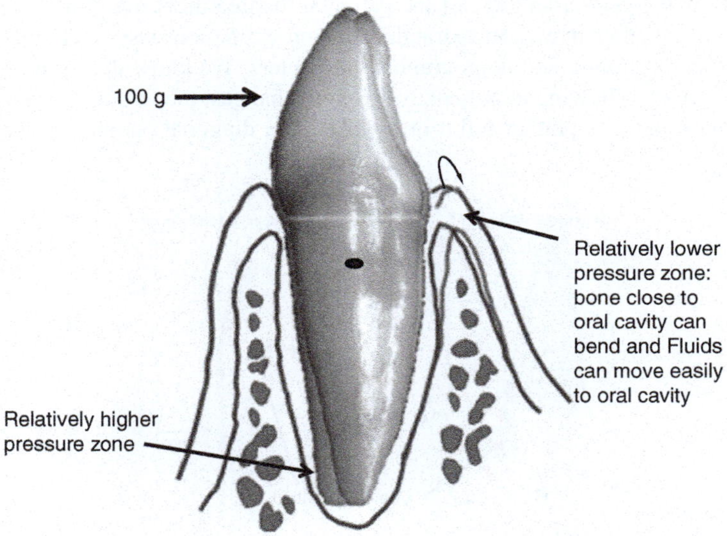

Fig. 4.6 High and low pressure along the root surface. When 100 g of force is applied to the crown, the root moves accordingly. Crestal bone can bend (decrease the pressure), while the apical bone cannot. Fluids from the crestal zone can easily move into the oral cavity (decrease the pressure) compared to the fluid in the apical zone. In most movements the stress in the apical zone exceeds the one on the gingival zone. Thus the pressure in the crestal zone can actually be decreased or is much lower than in the apical zone, and therefore it is rare to see the signs of root resorption in the gingival zone

Knowledge achieved from animal experiments, in which the researches were trying to imitate clinical human conditions, is important. However, there is always a risk of drawing conclusions from those experiments to humans. Human orthodontitis clinical studies are unfortunately short term in nature and usually examine the first premolars. Drawing clinical conclusions from 4- to 12-week studies on the behavior of the TPLBS exposed to 24 or more months of treatment is questionable. Moreover, the teeth that are examined in those studies, the first premolars, are usually the teeth that are not very susceptible and vulnerable to present signs of IDO. Further, we do not recall any short-term study where actual root shortening was reported. Therefore, it might be summarized that drawing long-term clinical conclusions from many laboratory studies is far from being accurate. We believe that similar attitude has to be toward studies using computer programs that simulate the actual conditions of the TPLBS. The finite element model (FEM) is the most popular one in this context [14, 79, 80, 154]. Although this engineering program accepts numerous physical properties' variables of the biological components, again, drawing conclusions on the human TPLBS is limited and has to be taken very carefully since it is impossible to follow the changes in time and of course to consider the individual variations in the reaction to force application.

This part of the review will present and discuss orthodontitis and the effect of different patient-related factors published in the last decade:

4.1 Genetic Factors

The present concept in the professional literature is that *bone* remodeling is controlled by inflammation process. The current assumption says that normal bone remodeling is a reaction to probably local micro-fractures or local fatigue areas of the bone. This process is genetically controlled [13]. The term "bone remodeling" means that at the end of the precise timing process, a full regeneration (functional and morphological) of the remodeled part is completed. Since the cementum is very comparable to the alveolar bone, the implication of the remodeling process from the bone to the cementum is logical, especially since it was shown that alveolar bone remodeling and physiological cemental remodeling are alike [155]. As mentioned before it might be that the cemental remodeling process is the outcome of IO; however in IDO the process goes beyond the cementum borders into the dentin to become irreversible minimodeling process (morphological root changes). Most of the current genetic research of the physiological (the one that is limited to the cementum) and the pathological (the one that damages the dentine) orthodontitis (IO and IDO) deals with parameters that are well known from the medical literature for being responsible to the inflammation process. Humoral and cell parameters like RANK, RANKL, OPG, P2X7R, cytokines, interleukins, prostaglandins, etc., and of course genetic expressions such as genotype, phenotype, polymorphism, and others are the main actors of the many research projects currently studying thoroughly the full extent of orthodontitis [14, 23–26, 35–41, 43, 128, 129].

We see the Harris et al. [141] and Al-Qawasami et al. [23] publications as the two milestones related to hereditary and orthodontitis. Harris' clinical research studied the meaning of patients' susceptibility to EARR. The conclusion of this article says: "Even when the nature of the malocclusion, the treatment plan, the appliance and the practitioner appear to be held constant there is a considerable range among patients, in the occurrence and the extent of EARR. One interpretation of these differences is that the person's genotype modulates his or her susceptibility to EARR: some people appear to be intrinsically endowed with resistance to apical resorption under the stress of mechanotherapy, and some, at the other extreme, are prone to experience severe resorption under the same regimen." This conclusion was challenged by the group from Indiana University who conducted their genetic-related studies for the last decade. The 2003 epic publication by this group was the first one to report on a genetic marker that identifies people who are susceptible to ORR before the beginning of orthodontic treatment. This research found association of EARR and IL-1β polymorphism suggesting a role of this cytokine in the pathogenesis of EARR. One of the conclusions of this article suggested that potential orthodontic patients can be screened for IL-1β genotype by analyzing the DNA from a simple cheek swab or mouthwash taken during initial examination to identify those who carry 2 copies of the high-risk allele (allele 1 of IL-1β). As of today, almost 10 years after this study was published, we are not aware of any clinic that does this test, nor did we read any prospective study that found potential orthodontic patients who carry two copies of this allele, and their susceptibility to EARR was evaluated during and following treatment. Further, another retrospective study [37] found that the allele and the genotype distribution of the IL-1β polymorphism in patients and control cohorts revealed no indication of a predisposition to EARR, and another group [26] found, with much higher logarithmic odds (LOD) score than the Al-Qawasmi et al. group [23], that variations in the interleukin 1-RN (IL-1 receptor antagonist) gene and not only in the IL-1β gene are determinants of a predisposition to postorthodontic EARR. The debate on the role of genetic polymorphism as well as different biologic agents like interleukins, prostaglandins, RANK and RANKL, osteoprotegrin (OPG) [40], TNFα, TNFRSF11A, TNSALP [35, 39], and others on the susceptibility to EARR is ongoing, and we hope that in the future it will be cleared and solved.

4.2 Immune System Factors

Surprisingly, the number of publications discussing role of the immune system in orthodontitis, in the last 20 years, is minute relative to the overwhelming number of publications related to genetics of the inflammation process and orthodontitis. As mentioned previously, this might be the effect of the shift of the current medical discourse to the genome role in physiological and pathological conditions.

It is well known that the immune reaction itself and the modulation of different lymphocytes response go mutually with the components of the inflammatory process [156, 157]. Therefore it might be just a question of time that this issue will become again a part of the medical discourse and the dental discourse as well. Years ago it was hypothesized that susceptibility to detrimental orthodontitis may be associated with autoimmune response to dentine matrix proteins [45, 158]. This was based on the evidence that anti-dentine antibodies could be detected in experimental root lesions in mice. The recent paper by Ramos et al. [46] concludes with two important issues that should get more attention:

(a) Each individual carries antibodies against the dentin matrix, which might not be recognized as a self-structure by the human immunologic system (probably from the time of the physiological exposure of the material during the replacement of the deciduous dentition). These antibodies may become active upon exposure of the dentin during the hyalinization that leads to damage of the cementum layer and dentine exposure. The level of these antibodies decreases during orthodontic treatment especially in patients who suffer from more extensive IDO [159].
(b) Relatively high levels of anti-human-dentine-extract (HDE) secretory IgA (sIgA) are simple indicators for patient's susceptibility to IDO. This antibody is the main line of defense of the oral cavity and the upper respiratory tract surfaces and is secreted in large amounts into the saliva by the salivary glands [128].

This study further suggests to analyze the level of this antibody (sIgA) before initiating orthodontic treatment in order to learn about the susceptibility of the patient to IDO, in a similar way to the study of Al-Qawasamy et al. [23], who suggested the DNA examination for two copies of allele 1 of IL-1β in new orthodontic patients.

4.3 Other Systemic Factors

The patient's systemic condition in relation to IDO continues to be investigated and is focused on two main issues. One is the spontaneous systemic state and the other one is the systemic status derived from influences of external factors: substances such as drugs, food supplements, hormones, and other materials and therapeutic procedures such as surgical. The systemic condition that involves no dispute regarding its influence on IDO is *allergy* including asthma.

Owman-Moll and Kurol [47] selected fifty adolescents and divided them into two equal groups: the high-risk group based on measurements of the most severe IDO, namely, IOD2 expression, and the low-risk group based on measurements of mild or no changes in root morphology IO and IDO1 expression. After a preliminary screening of possible risk factors regarding IDO, only subjects with allergy showed an increased risk of root resorption, but *this was without statistical significance*.

In 2006, Nishioka et al. [48] studied retrospectively the association between IDO2 expression and immune system factors in 60 Japanese orthodontic patients. The pretreatment records revealed that the incidence of allergy was significantly higher in the IDO2 group. The incidence of asthma also tended to be higher in this group. From these results, they concluded that allergy and asthma may be high-risk factors for the development of excessive root shortening during orthodontic tooth movement in Japanese patients.

Periodontitis was suggested to influence orthodontitis in a similar way to allergy and asthma as the number of inflammatory cells in the tissues adjacent to the roots of the teeth increases; however this issue was never studied or verified directly, and no conclusion related to ORR can be drawn. For example, experimental periodontitis was induced in rats by placing a cotton ligature around the cervix of the first upper molars for 48 h. An increase in the percentage of resorption areas and in the number of odontoclasts following orthodontic force application was found. These histomorphometric values were reduced once the inflammatory reaction had subsided. The results suggest delaying orthodontic treatment in patients with periodontal disease until the inflammatory signs have subsided [49]. Can we draw clinical conclusions from this 2-day rat experiment on the effect of periodontitis in conjunction with orthodontic force application to humans especially related to apical root shortening?

4.4 Chronologic Age

As most studies in previous decades found no significant correlation between the age of the orthodontic patients and the incidence and severity of IDO expression, it was quite surprising to find different results in recent studies. The results of a study in rats [65] revealed that adult rats (9–12 months old) had increased incidence and severity of root shortening with prolonged tooth movement compared to young rats (6 weeks old). In both groups, the middle part of the root had the highest incidence and severity of resorption. A clinical study by Jiang et al. [66] on 96 patients between 9 and 34 years treated by fixed appliances for at least 1 year found that patient age correlated with RR of the upper incisors before treatment and after treatment according to panoramic radiographs. It may be speculated that more ORR occurred in adults due to the presence of resorbed roots before treatment. However, the inaccuracy of analyzing the exact amount of ORR on panoramic radiographs is a well-known phenomenon [160, 161].

4.5 Dental Age

There is a consensus in the professional literature that ORR is related to the process of root development and that there is an advantage of moving teeth with incomplete root development regarding prevention of root shortening. However, while Hendrix et al. [47] found that teeth with incomplete root formation at the onset of orthodontic treatment continue to develop roots during treatment, but the roots reach somewhat less than their expected root length potential, Mavragani et al. [68] found no significant difference in the extent of root lengthening between the roots that elongated during treatment and the normal root lengthening in age-matched untreated individuals. They also found that roots that were incompletely developed before treatment reached a significantly greater length than those that were fully developed at the start of treatment. The differences between the two publications might be the result of the way the teeth were X-rayed and the roots' length was measured [159, 160].

4.6 Gender

All recent studies found no association between gender and IDO expression. No difference in either the incidence or severity of ORR between male and female patients was found in a study by Sameshima and Sinclair [69] who used periapical radiographs of 868 patients who were treated with full, fixed edgewise appliances. No statistically significant differences in ORR were found in relation to gender in a group of 96 subjects treated using fixed appliances for at least 1 year and who had panoramic radiographs at two time points [66]. "Even" the CBCT did not reveal a significant association between IDO and the gender of orthodontic patients [70].

4.7 Presence of RR Before and During Orthodontic Treatment

Confirmation to the positive correlation that was found in the past between the severity of ORR at the end of orthodontic treatment and the presence of ORR before treatment was given in the clinical study by Jiang et al. [66]. This correlation, obtained by evaluation of panoramic radiographs, was found especially for the anterior teeth.

Another correlation that was confirmed during the last decade by Artun et al. [71] is the positive correlation between the presence and severity of ORR during the initial stages of treatment and the severity of the resorption present at later stages, as evaluated on periapical radiographs for the maxillary central and lateral incisors. They found that patients with detectable ORR during the first 6 months of active treatment are more likely to experience resorption in the following 6-month period than those without. In a later study Artun et al. [72] found the amount of the resorption at the end of treatment to be highly correlated to that found after 6 and after 12 months of treatment.

4.8 Habits

Contrary to articles published in the past, the last published studies on the association between habits or parafunction on orthodontitis found no association. Owman-Moll and Kurol [47] checked the nail biting habit histologically on teeth that were moved orthodontically before their extractions, while Makedonas et al. [73] related to nail biting, nail biting history, finger sucking, and finger sucking history and used CBCT to evaluate the severity of resorption after 6 months of active treatment. They found no impact of the habits or past habits on the amount of the resorption.

4.9 Previously Traumatized Teeth

The only study in the last decade concerning OIRR in relation to previous trauma is the one by Makedonas et al. [73] who diagnosed ORR with CBCT after 6 months of orthodontic treatment with fixed appliances. The results of the study indicated that trauma before treatment did not have any impact on the amount of resorption after 6 months of active treatment.

4.10 Tooth Structure/Root Form

The different effect of the orthodontic force on teeth with different root forms is still in controversy. Some of the studies found root morphology as not being a risk factor for IDO [47, 70, 73, 76, 77]. Mavragani et al. [76] studied mild dental invagination and Van Parys et al. [77] pipette-shaped roots, and according to Lund et al. [70], root length at baseline was not associated with the degree of resorption. However, other studies reached different results. Smale et al. [78] report on long roots, narrow roots, and deviated root form as risk factors for EARR of the central incisors and on normal root form and wide roots as preventive factors. Nishioka et al. [48] found root morphology abnormality (shortened, blunt, eroded, pointed, bent, bottle shaped) significantly higher in the ORR group of orthodontically treated patients. Finite element model [79, 80] found various root morphologies affecting stress distribution of forces along the roots. Oyama et al. [79] applied forces in a vertical (intrusive) and horizontal (lingual) direction to the tooth axis and observed stress concentration in the root of the models with short, bent, and pipette-shaped roots. In the models with a bent or pipette-shaped root, significant stress was concentrated at the root apex. In the short-root model, significant stress was concentrated at the middle of the root, while the blunt-shaped root model showed no significant stress concentration at the root. Kamble et al. [80] applied orthodontic forces in various directions (intrusion, extrusion, tipping, and rotational) on maxillary central incisors and found significantly increased stress at the apex of the root with dilacerated morphology and at the cervical one-third region of the tooth with the short root. Increased stress was observed at the middle one-third region in the tooth with the pipette-shaped root during intrusion and extrusion. They conclude that the stress distribution pattern indicates that the maxillary central incisors with deviated root morphology are at higher risk of RR.

4.11 Topography of Adjacent Alveolar Bone

The bone factor regarding orthodontitis has been studied for decades. A study on tooth movement through regenerated bone created after distraction osteogenesis on beagles [81] found less resorption of the roots when the teeth were moved in mature, well-organized and mineralized bone created after 12 weeks of consolidation compared with immature, fibrous, and less-mineralized bone after 2 weeks of consolidation; however the amount of tooth movement was greater when the teeth were moved to immature bone although with more tipping. The effect of bone turnover rate on tooth movement and RR in rats was studied by inducing secondary hypo- and hyperthyroidism [82]. The different metabolic rates were created by this induction. It was found that low bone turnover induces a significantly larger amount of resorption on roots that are not submitted to mechanical loading. However the amount of RR induced by the orthodontic force was not influenced by the metabolic rate. The high bone turnover in the hyperthyroidism group increased the amount of orthodontic tooth movement but did not decrease the amount of IDO. It has to be noted again that administration of low doses of thyroid hormone (TH) was found to have a protective role on the root surface during orthodontic treatment [60]. Controversial reports on the association between alveolar bone density and orthodontitis appear in the literature [11]. Bone structure effect on orthodontitis of lower incisors was studied on pre- and posttreatment cephalometric radiographs of orthodontic patients by Otis [84]. No significant correlation was found between the extent of the IDO and the amount of alveolar bone around the root, the thickness of cortical bone, and the density of the trabecular network. Motokawa et al. [84] hypothesized that a movement of the maxillary central incisor near the cortical bone of the alveolus and incisive canal might cause severe RR.

4.12 Individual Tooth Susceptibility

All teeth may suffer from RR induced by the inflammation created by the orthodontic movement [11]; however several studies indicate that some of the teeth are more vulnerable to IDO than others. Apajalahti and Peltola [85] report that according to their study that used panoramic radiographs pre- and posttreatment, the most severe resorption was seen in the maxillary incisors and premolars. However according to most studies, the maxillary incisors are the most affected by RR during orthodontic treatment. This might be due to the greater movement of these teeth compared to other teeth during orthodontic treatment in order to achieve greater esthetic and functional demands [11] Mohandesan et al. [86] who studied the roots of maxillary incisors on periapical radiographs before and 6 and 12 months after the start of treatment found more shortening of the roots of the lateral incisors compared to those of the central incisors and that clinically significant resorption was found at a higher rate for the laterals compared to the centrals.

Opposite results were obtained recently by Jung and Cho [87] who report that according to their study on panoramic radiographs, maxillary central incisors were found to be the most resorbed teeth, followed by the maxillary lateral incisor. They found that the latter teeth are followed by the mandibular central incisors and the mandibular lateral incisors regarding vulnerability to IDO.

This part of the review will present and discuss the treatment-related factors affecting OIIRR published in the last decade:

4.13 Orthodontic Treatment-Related Factors

4.13.1 Force Magnitude

There is no orthodontic tooth movement without force application; therefore, the force level is the immediate or usual suspect blamed for IDO1 and IDO2. In the last decade, Darendeliler and his group in Sydney, Australia, published results of several researches using microcomputed tomography, scanning electron microscopy, and laser microscopy, discussing the force magnitude effect on orthodontitis [89–95]. In these studies, it was found that the volume of the resorption craters at least in certain areas of the roots (in human premolars and rats molars) was directly proportional to the force magnitude exerted for intrusion, extrusion, rotation, tipping, and bodily movements. Only one similar study, conducted by a group from the Netherlands [88] on mandibular premolars of dogs, that measured the dimensions of the lacunae found the effect of force magnitude on the severity of root resorption to be statistically insignificant. According to a recently published study by Darendeliler's group, when extremely heavy forces were applied on rats' molars, root resorption increased; however the amount of tooth movement decreased [89].

All those studies, which contributed tremendously to our understanding of the orthodontitis process, have to be taken with utmost care. Orthodontics human studies that involve extractions of teeth are usually short term. The average study length is a few months, while orthodontic treatment lasts usually 20–24 months. Moreover, the premolars which are the common teeth involved in those studies are not the ones that suffer from IDO1 and IDO2 as, for example, the upper incisors and none of the extracted teeth demonstrated apical RR. Again, we can learn a lot from animal studies; however the implication from those studies on human beings is not always correct and exact.

4.13.2 Duration of Force Application

No study to date contradicted the direct correlation found between the duration of force application and the severity and incidence/prevalence of the resorption that occurs during treatment, whether those studies were clinical [86, 96] or histological [88, 97, 98]. It is more than reasonable to assume that long-term exposure of the roots to orthodontitis might eventually lead to IDO1 or even to IDO2 expression. As we previously mentioned, genes and their products and the proteins act differently in changing environment; therefore, the longer the treatment, the chances of the environment to change increases.

4.13.3 Orthodontic Type of Movement

Teeth are probably more vulnerable to intrusion. It was found that applying intrusive 100 cN of continuous force to maxillary first human premolar teeth for 8 weeks prior to their extractions produced about four times more root resorption than similar extrusive force [99].

Moreover, other [100, 101] clinical studies found that movements combined with intrusion are more detrimental to the roots (IDO1 and IDO2) than nonintrusive mechanics.

These findings match others who found that significant resorption occurs more in compression areas compared to tension areas and can explain the findings that IDO1 and IDO2 expressions following tipping movement are more pronounced than that resulting from bodily movement as the pressure is dispersed along the roots in the last mentioned type of movement [89]. Unfortunately the effect of torque per se on the IDO1 and IDO2 expression was not studied in the last decade.

4.13.4 The Treatment Method

There is evidence that IDO1 and IDO2 manifestations are present in all forms and methods of treatment. The use of *removable thermoplastic appliances* does not prevent this side effect. Krieger E et al. [103] found that all 100 patients included in their study that were treated to resolve anterior crowding by aligners had a reduction of the pretreatment root length. According to a previous microcomputed tomography study by Barbagallo et al., clear removable thermoplastic appliances have, in a short term, in vivo experiment similar effects on root cementum as light (25 g) orthodontic forces derived from fixed appliances [104].

Also the use of *self-ligating brackets* does not reduce the incidence and severity of root uptake compared to the use of conventional brackets [105–107].

All the studies from the last decade that dealt with the effect of treatment involving extractions on IDO expression compared to treatment without extractions found that the first one resulted statistically significant higher prevalence of severe root resorption [84, 86, 108, 109] probably due to the distance of teeth and roots moved during treatment.

However, no difference was found in root resorption between two-step and en masse space closure procedures [110]. Even though the use of super-elastic heat-activated arch wires was not found to significantly increase the severity of root resorption, compared to conventional multi-stranded stainless steel arch wires during the leveling stage of treatment [111], most studies found that intermittent forces cause less severe root resorption than continuous forces [88, 112–114]. However there might be clinical importance to the timing of reactivation according to the last mentioned study.

A recent study found that more root resorption in patients is treated by the *straight-wire* method and less in the *standard edgewise* technique. The authors suggest that it may be attributed to more root movement in the pre-adjusted MBT technique that was used to represent the straight-wire method [115].

Corticotomy-*facilitated orthodontics* (CFO) in adults to relieve moderate crowding of the lower anterior teeth was found to reduce the total time of treatment significantly from 17.5 ± 2.8 weeks in the CFO group to 49 ± 12.3 weeks in the conventional orthodontic therapy group and decreasing the root length lost (0.02±0.10 mm compared to 1.4±0.8 mm) with no statistical significance [116]. No difference in the amount of resorption between the *Fränkel and eruption guidance appliance* groups was found [117].

The use of *magnets* for orthodontic tooth movements in rats by gradually increasing the force applied induced effective tooth movement with no pathological changes, such as root resorption [118]. However, this method has not been developed enough for clinical use.

A study by Brin et al. [162] that compared *1- versus 2-phase treatment* of class II malocclusion found the proportion of incisors with moderate to severe ORR to be slightly greater in the 1-phase treatment group.

4.14 Non-orthodontic Treatment-Related Factors

4.14.1 Endodontically Treated Teeth

Although in the past there was disagreement over the correlation between endodontically treated teeth and ORR [11], recent studies on periapical or panoramic radiographs indicate no significant difference in the amount or severity of RR during orthodontic treatment between root-filled teeth and teeth with vital pulps [74, 75, 120]. However a recent study found that genetic variations in the interleukin-1β gene predispose root-filled teeth to EARR for matched pairs, secondary to orthodontic treatment in a different way from their control teeth with vital pulps in subjects homozygous for allele 2 [2/2(TT)] [42].

Nonsteroid anti-inflammatory drugs (NSAID) are sometimes used to relieve pain during orthodontic tooth movement. Nabumetone given to orthodontic patients was found to be useful in reducing IDO manifestations, pulpitis, and pain caused by intrusive orthodontic movement, without altering tooth movement in response to the application of orthodontic force [50]. These results strengthen the inflammation base of orthodontitis.

Doxycycline is one of the tetracycline antibiotics group and is commonly used to treat a variety of infections including chronic ones. Mavragani et al. [51] investigated the effect of systemic administration of low-dose doxycycline on ORR in rats and found a significant reduction in ORR, in the number of odontoclasts, osteoclasts, mononuclear cells on the root surface, and TRAP-positive cells on the root and bone for the doxycycline-administered group. The effect of the doxycycline may be at least partly similar to that of the NSAIDs.

Bisphosphonates, known to be inhibitors of bone resorption, continued to be studied in relation to orthodontic tooth movement in the last decade probably due their vast use in treatment for bone metabolism disorders such as osteoporosis, Paget's disease, and bone metastases. While in the past there was a dispute over the effect of bisphosphonates on the roots during orthodontic movement, according to the studies of the last decade, these agents reduce ORR. The bisphosphonates inhibit the ability of osteoclasts to resorb bone by mechanisms that interfere with cytoskeletal organization and formation of the ruffled border, and this leads to cell death by apoptosis [52, 53]. Fujimura et al. [54] found in their study on mice that bisphosphonates reduced the amount of tooth movement and the number of osteoclasts. In addition, they also reduced ORR on the pressure side. Thus they concluded that bisphosphonates inhibit orthodontic tooth movement and prevent RR during orthodontic tooth movement in mice. Similar results were obtained earlier by Liu et al. [55] and later by Choi et al. [56], who found dose-dependent effect of the clodronate, a non-N-containing bisphosphonate or first-generation bisphosphonate, in rats. Their conclusion was that although clodronate might decrease RR related to orthodontic tooth movement, patients should be informed about a possible decrease in the amount of tooth movement and a prolonged period of orthodontic treatment.

According to a systematic review on the influence of bisphosphonates in orthodontic therapy that was published in 2010 [57], no data are available on the effect of longer than 21 days of bisphosphonates treatment, which is an important issue given the well-known side effects of this type of drug, which include maxillary osteonecrosis.

The apoptosis of osteoclasts that leads to reduction in bone and RR is in contradiction to the theory that reduced bone resorption increases RR [23].

Ovariectomy causes reduced estrogen levels resulting increased osteoclastogenesis [61]. Ovariectomy of female rats, performed to mimic postmenopausal patients, was found to affect tooth movement and orthodontitis. Tooth movement in the ovariectomy group was found to be more rapid and the amount of root shortening was more severe than in a control group [62]. A recent study [63] found that treatment of ovariectomized rats by systemic zoledronic acid, a potent and novel bisphosphonate that is used for the treatment of osteoporosis, inhibits orthodontic tooth movement and also reduces the risk of IDO2 expression in the ovariectomized rats. The mechanisms of action and the pharmacologic properties of the zoledronic acid directly involve the induction of osteoclast apoptosis [64]. These studies, albeit in rats, raise the awareness of the differences we may expect in treating orthodontically postmenopausal women.

4.14.2 Sympathectomy

Haug et al. [121] found that sympathectomized (SCGx) rats had significantly more RR and substance P-immunoreactive fibers in the compressed periodontal ligament following orthodontic tooth movement compared with control rats. This publication demonstrates that there might be a direct connection between orthodontitis and the nervous system, in this case the sympathetic one. We hope that the research of those relationships will be studied in the future.

4.14.3 Fluoride

The effects of fluoride intake on the roots during orthodontic tooth movement began to be explored on rats by Australian groups led by Darendeliler in the last decade. In 2007 it was reported that fluoride reduces the size of resorption craters, but the effect is variable and not statistically significant ($P>.05$) [58]. In 2011 the findings were that RR lesions of the group exposed to fluoride were significantly reduced in length and depth ($P<0.01$) [12]. The mineral content of the RR craters of the fluoride group had higher concentrations of fluorine and zinc ($P<0.01$). There was less calcium in the craters of the no-fluoride group compared with the fluoride group ($P<0.05$). The conclusion was that cementum quality (influenced by systemic fluoride exposure) might impact the extent of orthodontically induced resorptive defects. Another study of the group [59] found that fluoride reduced the depth, volume, and roughness of the resorption craters in the experimental groups. Regarding the duration of fluoride intake, it was found that the longer fluoride was administered via drinking water to the rats since their birth, the smaller the amount of tooth movement observed. Their conclusion was that fluoride in drinking water from birth reduced the severity of OIRR, but the amount of tooth movement was also decreased. The author's hypotheses as to the action of fluoride are that fluoride could suppress RR by similar mechanisms present in caries: acid resistance, enhancement of remineralization, and suppression of odontoclasts. However, according to the last study of the group regarding fluoride effect on roots of patients, a high fluoride intake from public water did not have a beneficial effect on the severity of root resorption after a 4-week orthodontic force application and 12 weeks of passive retention [163].

4.14.4 Thyroid Hormone

The protective effect of thyroid hormone administration was confirmed by Vázquez-Landaverde et al. [60] who studied the effect of thyroid hormone-treated rats (intraperitoneal and oral) during orthodontic tooth movement. Circulating T3 levels, systemic alkaline phosphatase (APase) activity, and 5′deiodinase (5′D) activity were evaluated in the periodontal area. The results showed that TH-treated animals (intraperitoneal or oral) had significantly less force-induced root resorptive lesions compared with a control group, without apparent changes in T3 or alkaline phosphatase levels, and that periodontal remodeling was accompanied by a significant increase in local T3 generation as a result of T4 deiodination. This 5′D activity was higher in those animals that received exogenous TH. These results suggest that this protective TH mechanism may be achieved at a local level and that administration of low doses of TH may play a protective role on the root surface.

4.14.5 Light-Emitting Diode (LED) Therapy

The effects of light-emitting diode (LED) therapy at 940 nm on inflammatory RR were studied in rats. Animals submitted to orthodontic force plus LED therapy presented significantly fewer osteoclasts and inflammatory cells and more blood vessels and fibroblasts in the periodontal ligament than the non-irradiated animals. The results led the authors to suggest that LED therapy may improve periodontal tissue repair and decrease inflammation and RR after the application of orthodontic force [122].

4.14.6 Ultrasound

El-Bialy et al. [124] evaluated the effect of low-intensity pulsed ultrasound (LIPUS) known to enhance healing of traumatized connective tissues with IDO expression in humans. Histological examination revealed healing of the resorbed root surface by hypercementosis, and the scanning electron microscopy (SEM) study showed a statistically significant decrease in the areas of resorption and the number of resorption lacunae in the LIPUS-exposed premolars.

A study on rats found that LIPUS enhances repair of IDO damages by decreasing the number of osteoclasts and their level of activity probably as a result of increasing the ratio osteoprotegerin (OPT) to the receptor activator of nuclear factor kappa-B ligand (RANKL). Reparative cementum was found in the LIPUS-treated samples of rats by means of high-power SEM [123].

Similar results were obtained by a recent study [164] that expects LIPUS to be applicable to clinical use in the near future.

4.15 In Summary

Orthodontitis is the inflammation that involves the periodontal ligament, bone, cementum, and many times the dentine. It is the direct result of orthodontic force application that initiates a sequential genetic-environmental cellular process. This inflammation is the biological process that is behind every tooth movement and might lead to minor (IO) up to severe manifestations of root resorption (IDO1 or IDO2). We know exactly how and when it evokes, but until today, we are unable to predict its overall outcome that goes beyond the desirable tooth movement into unwanted resorption of the roots (IDO1 and IDO2 expression). The intensity and the length of the inflammatory process depend on many factors. Some of them are genetically related (*patient related*, personal vulnerability, or personal susceptibility), while others are *treatment related* (orthodontic and non-orthodontic), and most of them are still, even after the human genome was decoded, beyond our knowledge. This inflammation is physiologically or normally responsible for bone as well as cemental remodeling; however, for yet unknown reasons there might be a failure in the coupling process, which let the resorption continue beyond the borders of the cementum into the dentin. Unfortunately, this tissue cannot regenerate since the dentinoblasts are in the pulp and not in the dentino-cemental junction. When the damage is large enough, the morphological changes can be detected using external imaging techniques. From the three tissues involved in orthodontitis, the periodontal ligament and the bone, both are fully regenerated, while the root is not.

This review presents the readers a new term – orthodontitis – and also suggests three theories to the understanding of the process:

(a) Reaction of the body to unrecognized extreme new conditions
(b) Hidden part of the evolutionary process – the tissue hierarchy theory
(c) Orthodontitis as a self-defense mechanism

Most of the publications quoted in this review draw their legitimacy from knowledge extracted out of evidence-based dentistry studies; however some publications can be defined as "expectation-based dentistry," since their outcome has not been challenged yet.

Appendix

Suggested protocol to minimize orthodontic root resorption (ORR) and to avoid periodontitis consequences during orthodontic treatment (OT) for new and earlier orthodontic-treated patients. Orthodontitis and its consequences should be a part of any orthodontic treatment informed consent (Brezniak and Wasserstein 2016):

Orthodontitis and its unwanted ORR results as well as different types of periodontitis must be discussed with the patients/parents/guardians prior to the treatment and when positive findings were revealed during and following OT. This protocol is only a general suggestion or general guidelines and it does not replace the orthodontist' professional medical discretion/judgment and responsibility of the consequences during and following OT.

Definitions

Monitoring: PA X-ray of the upper incisors

Standard Monitoring (SM): Monitoring following 9–12 months of force application to the incisors and at least once a year in a lengthy treatment

Frequent Monitoring (FM): Monitoring every 6–9 months following force activation on the incisors

Intensive Monitoring (IM): Monitoring every 4–6 months following force activation on the incisors

I. General health – Does the patient suffer from allergy[1]? If yes use FM protocol.
II. Dental health – Does the patient suffer from periodontitis? If yes send the patient to the periodontist to discuss further related treatment considerations. When treatment lasts, use IM protocol adding bitewing X-ray every 4–6 months.
    A. New patient before treatment:
        1. Does the patient have signs of RR (idiopathic, tooth related, etc.)? Go to 3b.
        2. Does the patient demonstrate any periodontal problem (loss of bone support, cervical resorption, etc.)? If yes, go to II.
        3. Was a close family member of the patient orthodontically treated in the past?

[1]Allergy symbolizes many other systemic medical conditions that most of them including allergy have controversial relationship to orthodontitis and its manifestations.

   (a) Was ORR detected? If not use SM protocol.
   (b) Is the amount of ORR on PA film:
      1. Less than 2 mm? Use SM during treatment.
      2. More than 2 mm but less than 1/3 of the root? Use FM protocol during treatment. Initiate treatment without extraction if needed, and decide only following 4–6 months in treatment.
      3. More than 1/3 of the root? Use 3b2 protocol; however use IM protocol during treatment.

B. An earlier treated orthodontic patient or a transfer patient:
   1. Does the patient have signs of ORR on a mandatory incisors' PA film? If not use SM; otherwise use 3b protocol.
   2. Does the patient have signs of periodontal disease on mandatory incisors' PA film and/or bitewing X-rays? If yes send the patient to the periodontist to discuss further related treatment considerations. Use FM protocol as well as bitewing X-rays every 4–6 months.

C. Monitoring findings during treatment:
   1. Does the patient have signs of ORR? If not continue to use SM; otherwise:
      (a) Less than 2 mm? Use FM during further treatment.
      (b) More than 2 mm but less than 1/3 of the root? Pause the treatment for 2–3 months. Take a new radiograph following 3 months in re-treatment to re-evaluate treatment continuation.
      (c) More than 1/3 of the root? Pause the treatment for 2–3 months. Further treatment procedures depend on the current conditions:
         1. If close to the finish – Do as much as you can to finish treatment in a short time with compromises if needed. Try to avoid torque movements as much as you can. Use IM during treatment.
         2. If more than a year estimated to finish – Change treatment goals; change treatment modalities like using TADS as anchorage; evaluate surgical procedures; consider implants in extraction spaces if possible and if needed; avoid using resorbed teeth as anchored ones; don't use rectangular wires and avoid torque movements. Use IM during treatment.
   2. Does the patient have signs of periodontal disease on PA or bitewing X-ray? If yes go to II.

D. Findings following treatment:
   1. Any type of ORR and/or periodontal disease should be discussed thoroughly with the patients/parents/guardians.
   2. Teeth with mild or even severe ORR should rarely if ever be extracted. Fixed retention (sometimes double retention) attached to non-damaged teeth or fused bridges are the best long-term solution suggested for extreme cases.

References

1. Bletsa A, Berggreen E, Brudvik P. Interleukin-1alpha and tumor necrosis factor-alpha expression during the early phases of orthodontic tooth movement in rats. Eur J Oral Sci. 2006;114:423–9.
2. Garlet TP, Coelho U, Silva JS, Garlet GP. Cytokine expression pattern in compression and tension sides of the periodontal ligament during orthodontic tooth movement in humans. Eur J Oral Sci. 2007;115:355–62.
3. Tzannetou S, Efstratiadis S, Nicolay O, Grbic J, Lamster I. Comparison of levels of inflammatory mediators IL-1beta and betaG in gingival crevicular fluid from molars, premolars, and incisors during rapid palatal expansion. Am J Orthod Dentofacial Orthop. 2008;133:699–707.
4. Surlin P, Rauten AM, Silosi I, Foia L. Pentraxin-3 levels in gingival crevicular fluid during orthodontic tooth movement in young and adult patients. Angle Orthod. 2012;82:833–8.
5. Kim SJ, Park KH, Park YG, Lee SW, Kang YG. Compressive stress induced the up-regulation of M-CSF, RANKL, TNF-α expression and the down-regulation of OPG expression in PDL cells via the integrin-FAK pathway. Arch Oral Biol. 2013;58:707–16.
6. Brezniak N, Wasserstein A. Orthodonticall induced inflammatory root resorption. Part 1: the basic science aspects. Angle Orthod. 2002;72(2):175–9.
7. Brezniak N, Wasserstein A. Orthodonticall induced inflammatory root resorption. Part II: the clinical aspects. Angle Orthod. 2002;72(2):180–4.
8. Brudvik P, Rygh P. Transition and determinants of orthodontic root resorption-repair sequence. Eur J Orthod. 1995;17(3):177–88.
9. Brezniak N, Wasserstein A. Defining and framing orthodontitis: a new term in orthodontics. Angle Orthod. 2014;84(3):568–9.
10. www.merriam-webster.com. www.merriam-webster.com. [Online] [Cited: Dec 2014.] http://www.merriam-webster.com/medical/itis.
11. Brezniak N, Wasserstein A. Root resorption after orthodontic treatment: part 1. Am J Orthod Dentofacial Orthop. 1993;103(1):62–6.
12. Gonzales C, Hotokezaka H, Karadeniz EI, Miyazaki T, Kobayashi E, Darendeliler MA, Yoshida N. Effects of fluoride intake on orthodontic tooth movement and orthodontically induced root resorption. Am J Orthod Dentofacial Orthop. 2011;139(2):196–205.
13. Roberts WE. In: Vanarsdall RL Jr, Vig KWJ, Graber LW, editors. Bone Physiology, Metabolism, and Biomechanics in Orthodontic Treatment Phliadelphia. 5th ed. s. l. Mosby; 2012. p. 386–453.
14. Viecilli RF, Katona TR, Chen J, Hartsfield Jr JK, Roberts WE. Orthodontic mechanotransduction and the role of the P2X7 receptor. Am J Orthod Dentofacial Orthop. 2009;135(6):694.e1–16.
15. Brudvik P, Rygh P. The initial phase of orthodontic root resorption incident to local compression of the periodontal ligament. Eur J Orthod. 1993;15:249–63.
16. Andreasen JO. Review of root resorption systems and models. In: Davidivitch Z, editor. The Biological Mechanisms of Tooth Eruption and Root Resorption. EBSCO Media, Birmingham, AL, 1988. p. 9–22.
17. Malcolm J, Clement C. The pain and discomfort experienced during orthodontic treatment: A randomized controlled clinical trial of two intial aligning arch wires. Am J Orthod. 1992;102(4):373–81.
18. Tanaka E, Ueki K, Kikuzaki M, Yamada E, Takeuchi M, Dalla-Bona D, Tanne K. Longitudinal measurements of tooth mobility during orthodontic treatment using a periotest. Angle Orthod. 2005;75(1):101–5.
19. Hammad SM, El-Hawary YM, El-Hawary AK. The use of different analgesics in orthodontic tooth movements. Angle Orthod. 2012;82(5):820–6.
20. Levander E, Malmgren O. Evaluation of the risk of root resorption during orthodontic treatment: a study of upper incisors. Eur J Orthod. 1988;10(1):30–8.

21. Becker A, Chaushu S. Long-term follow-up of severely resorbed maxillary incisors after resolution of an etiologically associated impacted canine. Am J Orthod Dentofacial Orthop. 2005;127(6):650–4.
22. Marques LS, Chaves KC, Rey AC, Pereira LJ, Ruellas AC. Severe root resorption and orthodontic treatment: clinical implications after 25 years of follow-up. Am J Orthod Dentofacial Orthop. 2011;139(4 Suppl):S166–9.
23. Al-Qawasami RA, Hartsfield Jr JK, Everette ET, Flury L, Liu L, Foroud TM, Marci J, Roberts WE. Genetic predisposition to external apical root resorption. Am J Orthod Dentofacial Orthop. 2003;123(3):242–52.
24. Low E, Zoellner H, Kharbanda OP, Darendeliler MA. Expression of mRNA for osteoprotegerin and receptor activator of nuclear factor kappa beta ligand (RANKL) during root resorption induced by the application of heavy orthodontic forces on rat molars. Am J Orthod Dentofacial Orthop. 2005;128(4):497–503.
25. Bastos Lages EM, Drummond AF, Pretti H, Costa FO, Lages EJ, Gontijo AI, Miranda Cota LO, Brito Jr RB. Association of functional gene polymorphism IL-1beta in patients with external apical root resorption. Am J Orthod Dentofacial Orthop. 2009;136(4):542–6.
26. Iglesias-Linares A, Yañez-Vico R, Ballesta-Mudarra S, Ortiz-Ariza E, Ortega-Rivera H, Mendoza-Mendoza A, Solano-Reina E, Perea-Pérez E. Postorthodontic external root resorption is associated with IL1 receptor antagonist gene variations. Oral Dis. 2012;18(2):198–205.
27. Bates S. Absorption. Br J Dent Sci. 1856;1:256.
28. Ottolengui R. The physiological and pathological resorption of tooth roots. Items Interest. 1914;36:332–6.
29. Ketcham AH. A preliminary report of an investigation of apical root resorption of vital permanent teeth. Int J Orthod. 1927;13:97–127.
30. Collins FS, Morgan M, Patrinos A. The human genome project: lessons from large-scale biology. Science. 2003;300:286–90.
31. Linge BO, Linge L. Apicak root resorption in upper anterior teeth. Eur J Orthod. 1983;5:173–83.
32. Parker JR, Harris EF. Directions of orthodontic tooth movements associated with external apical root resorption of the maxillary central incisor. Am J Orthod Dentofacial Orthop. 1998;114(6):677–83.
33. Owman-Moll P, Kurol J, Lundgren D. Repair of orthodontically induced root resorption in adolescents. Angle Orthod. 1995;66(6):403–8.
34. Weltman B, Vig KW, Fields HW, Shanker S, Kaizar EE. Root resorption associated with orthodontic tooth movement: a systematic review. Am J Orthod Dentofacial Orthop. 2010;137(4):462–74.
35. Al-Qawasmi RA, Hartsfield Jr JK, Everett ET, Weaver MR, Foroud TM, Faust DM, Roberts WE. Root resorption associated with orthodontic force in inbred mice: genetic contributions. Eur J Orthod. 2006;28(1):13–9.
36. Abass SK, Hartsfield Jr JK, Al-Qawasmi RA, Everett ET, Foroud TM, Roberts WE. Inheritance of susceptibility to root resorption associated with orthodontic force in mice. Am J Orthod Dentofacial Orthop. 2008;134(6):472–750.
37. Gülden N, Eggermann T, Zerres K, Beer M, Meinelt A, Diedrich P. Interleukin-1 polymorphisms in relation to external apical root resorption (EARR). J Orofac Orthop. 2009;70(1):20–38.
38. Sehr K, Bock NC, Serbesis C, Hönemann M, Ruf S. Severe external apical root resorption – local cause or genetic predisposition? J Orofac Orthop. 2011;72(4):321–31.
39. Al-Qawasmi RA, Hartsfield Jr JK, Everett ET, Weaver MR, Foroud TM, Faust DM, Roberts WE. Root resorption associated with orthodontic force in IL-1B Knockout mouse. J Misculoskel Neuron Interact. 2004;4:383–5.
40. Zhao N, Liu Y, Kanzaki H, Liang W, Ni J, Lin J. Effects of local osteoprotegerin gene transfection on orthodontic root resorption during retention: an in vivo micro-CT analysis. Orthod Craniofac Res. 2012;15(1):10–20.

41. Hartsfield JK. Pathways in external apical root resorption associated with orthodontia. Orthod Craniofac Res. 2009;12(3):236–42.
42. Iglesias-Linares A, Yañez-Vico RM, Ballesta S, Ortiz-Ariza E, Mendoza-Mendoza A, Perea E, Solano-Reina E. Interleukin 1 gene cluster SNPs (rs1800587, rs1143634) influences post-orthodontic root resorption in endodontic and their contralateral vital control teeth differently. Int Endod J. 2012;45(11):108–26. doi:10.1111/j.1365-2591.2012.02065.x.
43. Wu FL, Wang LY, Huang YQ, Guo WB, Liu CD, Li SG. Interleukin-1β +3954 polymorphisms and risk of external apical root resorption in orthodontic treatment: a meta-analysis. Genet Mol Res. 2013;12(4):4678–86.
44. Silva LB, Guimaraes CS, Santos RA. Immunology of root resorption: a literature review. Indian J Dent Res. 2008;19(4):340–3.
45. Ng KT, King GJ, Courts FJ. Humoral immune response to active root resorption with a murine model. Am J Orthod Dentofacial Orthop. 1990;98(2):456–62.
46. de Ramos SP, Ortolan GO, Dos Santos LM, Tobouti PL, Hidalgo MM, Consolaro A, Itano EN. Anti-dentine antibodies with root resorption during orthodontic treatment. Eur J Orthod. 2011;33(5):584–91.
47. Owman-Moll P, Kurol J. Root resorption after orthodontic treatment in high- and low-risk patients: analysis of allergy as a possible predisposing factor. Eur J Orthod. 2000;22(6):657–63.
48. Nishioka M, Ioi H, Nakata S, Nakasima A, Counts A. Root resorption and immune system factors in the Japanese. Angle Orthod. 2006;76(1):103–8.
49. Garat JA, Martín AE, Gordillo ME, Ubios AM. Effect of orthodontic forces on root resorption in molars submitted to experimental periodontitis. Acta Odontol Latinoam. 2004;17(1–2):3–7.
50. Villa PA, Oberti G, Moncada CA, Vasseur O, Jaramillo A, Tobón D, Agudelo JA. Pulp-dentine complex changes and root resorption during intrusive orthodontic tooth movement in patients prescribed nabumetone. J Endod. 2005;31(1):61–6.
51. Mavragani M, Brudvik P, Selvig KA. Orthodontically induced root and alveolar bone resorption: inhibitory effect of systemic doxycycline administration in rats. Eur J Orthod. 2005;27(3):215–25.
52. Rogers MJ. New insights into the molecular mechanisms of action of bisphosphonates. Curr Pharm Des. 2003;9:2643–58.
53. Roelofs AJ, Thompson K, Gordon S, Rogers MJ. Molecular mechanisms of action of bisphosphonates: current status. Clin Cancer Res. 2006;12:6222s–30s.
54. Fujimura Y, Kitaura H, Yoshimatsu M, Eguchi T, Kohara H, Morita Y, Yoshida N. Influence of bisphosphonates on orthodontic tooth movement in mice. Eur J Orthod. 2009;31(6): 572–7.
55. Liu L, Igarashi K, Haruyama N, Saeki S, Shinoda H, Mitani H. Effects of local administration of clodronate on orthodontic tooth movement and root resorption in rats. Eur J Orthod. 2004;26(5):469–73.
56. Choi J, Baek SH, Lee JI, Chang YI. Effects of clodronate on early alveolar bone remodeling and root resorption related to orthodontic forces: a histomorphometric analysis. Am J Orthod Dentofacial Orthop. 2010;138(5):548e1–8.
57. Iglesias-Linares A, Yáñez-Vico RM, Solano-Reina E, Torres-Lagares D, González Moles MA. Influence of bisphosphonates in orthodontic therapy: systematic review. J Dent. 2010;38(8):603–11.
58. Foo M, Jones A, Darendeliler MA. Physical properties of root cementum: part 9. Effect of systemic fluoride intake on root resorption in rats. Am J Orthod Dentofacial Orthop. 2007;131(1):34–43.
59. Lim E, Belton D, Petocz P, Arora M, Cheng LL, Darendeliler MA. Physical properties of root cementum: part 15. Analysis of elemental composition by using proton-induced x-ray and gamma-ray emissions in orthodontically induced root resorption craters of rat molar cementum after exposure to systemic fluoride. Am J Orthod Dentofacial Orthop. 2011;139(2):e193–202.

60. Vázquez-Landaverde LA, Rojas-Huidobro R, Alonso Gallegos-Corona M, Aceves C. Periodontal 5′-deiodination on forced-induced root resorption – the protective effect of thyroid hormone administration. Eur J Orthod. 2004;24(4):363–9.
61. Horowitz MC. Cytokines and estrogen in bone: anti-osteoporotic effects. Science. 1993;260(5108):626–7.
62. Sirisoontorn I, Hotokezaka H, Hashimoto M, Gonzales C, Luppanapornlarp S, Darendeliler MA, Yoshida N. Tooth movement and root resorption; the effect of ovariectomy on orthodontic force application in rats. Angle Orthod. 2011;81(4):570–7.
63. Sirisoontorn I, Hotokezaka H, Hashimoto M, Gonzales C, Luppanapornlarp S, Darendeliler MA, Yoshida N. Orthodontic tooth movement and root resorption in ovariectomized rats treated by systemic administration of zoledronic acid. Am J Orthod Dentofacial Orthop. 2012;141(5):563–73.
64. Green JR. Bisphosphonates: preclinical review. Oncologist. 2004;9(Suppl):3–13.
65. Ren Y, Maltha JC, Liem RS, Stokroos I, Kuijpers-Jagtman AM. Age-dependent external root resorption during tooth movement in rats. Acta Odontol Scand. 2008;66(2):93–8.
66. Jiang RP, McDonald JP, Fu MK. Root resorption before and after orthodontic treatment: a clinical study of contributory factors. Eur J Orthod. 2010;32(6):693–7.
67. Hendrix I, Carels C, Kuijpers-Jagtman AM, Van'T Hof M. A radiographic study of posterior apical root resorption in orthodontic patients. Am J Orthod Dentofacial Orthop. 1994;105(4):345–9.
68. Mavragani M, Bøe OE, Wisth PJ, Selvig KA. Changes in root length during orthodontic treatment: advantages for immature teeth. Eur J Orthod. 2002;24(1):91–7.
69. Sameshima GT, Sinclair PM. Predicting and preventing root resorption: part I. Diagnostic factors. Am J Orthod Dentofacial Orthop. 2001;119(5):505–10.
70. Lund H, Gröndahl K, Hansen K, Gröndahl HG. Apical root resorption during orthodontic treatment. A prospective study using cone beam CT. Angle Orthod. 2012;82(3):480–7.
71. Artun J, Smale I, Behbehani F, Doppel D, Van't Hof M, Kuijpers-Jagtman AM. Apical root resorption six and 12 months after initiation of fixed orthodontic appliance therapy. Angle Orthod. 2005;75:919–26.
72. Artun J, Van't Hullenaar R, Doppel D, Kuijpers-Jagtman AM. Identification of orthodontic patients at risk of severe apical root resorption. Am J Orthod Dentofacial Orthop. 2009;135(4):448–55.
73. Makedonas D, Lund H, Gröndahl K, Hansen K. Root resorption diagnosed with cone beam computed tomography after 6 months of orthodontic treatment with fixed appliance and the relation to risk factors. Angle Orthod. 2012;82(2):196–201.
74. Llamas-Carreras JM, Amarilla A, Solano E, Velasco-Ortega E, Rodríguez-Varo L, Segura-Egea JJ. Study of external root resorption during orthodontic treatment in root filled teeth compared with their contralateral teeth with vital pulps. Am J Orthod Dentofacial Orthop. 1993;103(2):138–46.
75. Llamas-Carreras JM, Amarilla A, Espinar-Escalona E, Castellanos-Cosano L, Martín-González J, Sánchez-Domínguez B, López-Frías FJ. External apical root resorption in maxillary root-filled incisors after orthodontic treatment: a split-mouth design study. Med Oral Patol Oral Cir Bucal. 2012;17(3):e523–527.
76. Mavragani M, Apisariyakul J, Brudvik P, Selvig KA. Is mild dental invagination a risk factor for apical root resorption in orthodontic patients? Eur J Orthod. 2006;28(4):307–12.
77. Van Parys K, Aartman IH, Kuitert R, Zentner A. Relationship between dental anomalies and orthodontic root resorption of upper incisors. Eur J Orthod. 2012;34(5):571–4.
78. Smale I, Artun J, Behbehani F, Doppel D, van't Hof M, Kuijpers-Jagtman AM. Apical root resorption 6 months after initiation of fixed orthodontic appliance therapy. Am J Orthod Dentofacial Orthop. 2005;128(1):57–67.
79. Oyama K, Motoyoshi M, Hirabayashi M, Hosoi K, Shimizu N. Effects of root morphology on stress distribution at the root apex. Eur J Orthod. 2007;29(2):113–7.
80. Kamble RH, Lohkare S, Hararey PV, Mundada RD. Stress distribution pattern in a root of maxillary central incisor having various root morphologies. Angle Orthod. 2012;82(5):799–805.

81. Nakamoto N, Nagasaka H, Daimaruya T, Takahashi I, Sugawara J, Mitani H. Experimental tooth movement through mature and immature bone regenerates after distraction osteogenesis in dogs. Am J Orthod Dentofacial Orthop. 2002;121(4):385–95.
82. Verna C, Dalstra M, Melsen B. Bone turnover rate in rats does not influence root resorption induced by orthodontic treatment. Eur J Orthod. 2003;25(4):359–63.
83. Otis LL, Hong JS, Tuncay OC. Bone structure effect on root resorption. Orthod Craniofac Res. 2004;7(3):165–77.
84. Motokawa M, Sasamoto T, Kaku M, Kawata T, Matsuda Y, Terao A, Tanne K. Association between root resorption incident to orthodontic treatment and treatment factors. Eur J Orthod. 2012;34(3):350–6. Advance Access doi:10.1093/ejo/cjr018.
85. Apajalahti S, Peltola JS. Apical root resorption after orthodontic treatment – a retrospective study. Eur J Orthod. 2007;29(4):408–12.
86. Mohandesan H, Ravanmehr H, Valaei N. A radiographic analysis of external apical root resorption of maxillary incisors during active orthodontic treatment. Eur J Orthod. 2007;29(2):134–9.
87. Jung YH, Cho BH. External root resorption after orthodontic treatment: a study of contributing factors. Imaging Sci Dent. 2011;41(1):17–21.
88. Maltha JC, van Leeuwen EJ, Dijkman GE, Kuijpers-Jagtman AM. Incidence and severity of root resorption in orthodontically moved premolars in dogs. Orthod Craniofac Res. 2004;7(2):115–21.
89. Nakano T, Hotokezaka H, Hashimoto M, Sirisoontorn I, Arita K, Kurohama T, Darendeliler MA, Yoshida N. Effects of different types of tooth movement and force magnitudes on the amount of tooth movement and root resorption in rats. Angle Orthod. 2014;84(6):1079–85.
90. Montenegro VC, Jones A, Petocz P, Gonzales C, Darendeliler MA. Physical properties of root cementum: part 22. Root resorption after the application of light and heavy extrusive orthodontic forces: a microcomputed tomography study. Am J Orthod Dentofacial Orthop. 2012;141(1):1–9.
91. Wu AT, Turk T, Colak C, Elekdağ-Turk S, Jones AS, Petocz P, Darendeliler MA. Physical properties of root cementum: part 18. The extent of root resorption after the application of light and heavy controlled rotational orthodontic forces for 4 weeks: a microcomputed tomography. Am J Orthod Dentofacial Orthop. 2011;139(5):495–503.
92. Paetyangkul A, Türk T, Elekdağ-Türk S, Jones AS, Petocz P, Darendeliler MA. Physical properties of root cementum: part 14. The amount of root resorption after force application for 12 weeks on maxillary and mandibular premolars: a microcomputed-tomography study. Am J Orthod Dentofacial Orthop. 2009;136(4):492–9.
93. Harris DA, Jones AS, Darendeliler MA. Physical properties of root cementum: part 8. Volumetric analysis of root resorption craters after application of controlled intrusive light and heavy orthodontic forces: a microcomputed tomography scan study. Am J Orthod Dentofacial Orthop. 2006;130(5):639–47.
94. Chan E, Darendeliler MA. Physical properties of root cementum: part 5. Volumetric analysis of root resorption craters after application of light and heavy orthodontic forces. Am J Orthod Dentofacial Orthop. 2005;127(2):186–95.
95. Darnedeliler MA, Kharbanda OP, Chan EK, Srivicharnkul P, Rex T, Swain MV, Jones AS, Petocz P. Root resorption and its association with alterations in physical properties, mineral contents and resorption craters in human premolars following application of light and heavy controlled orthodontic forces. Orthod Craniofac Res. 2004;7(2):79–97.
96. Sameshima GT, Sinclair PM. Predicting and preventing root resorption: part II. Treatment factors. Am J Orthod Dentofacial Orthop. 2001;119(5):511–5.
97. Gonzales C, Hotokezaka H, Yoshimatsu M, Yozgatian JH, Darendeliler MA, Yoshida N. Force magnitude and duration effects on amount of tooth movement and root resorption in the rat molar. Angle Orthod. 2008;78(3):502–9.
98. Paetyangkul A, Türk T, Elekdağ-Türk S, Jones AS, Petocz P, Cheng LL, Darendeliler MA. Physical properties of root cementum: part 16. Comparisons of root resorption and resorption craters after the application of light and heavy continuous and controlled orthodontic forces for 4, 8, and 12 weeks. Am J Orthod Dentofacial Orthop. 2011;139(3):279–84.

99. Han G, Huang S, Von den Hoff JW, Zeng X, Kuijpers-Jagtman AM. Root resorption after orthodontic intrusion and extrusion: an intraindividual study. Angle Orthod. 2005;75(6):912–8.
100. Chiqueto K, Martins DR, Janson G. Effects of accentuated and reversed curve of Spee on apical root resorption. Am J Orthod Dentofacial Orthop. 2008;133(2):261–8.
101. Martins DR, Tibola D, Janson G, Maria FR. Effects of intrusion combined with anterior retraction on apical root resorption. Eur J Orthod. 2012;34(2):170–5.
102. Brezniak N, Wasserstein A. Root resorption following treatment with aligners. Angle Orthod. 2008;78(5):1119–24.
103. Krieger E, Drechsler T, Schmidtmann I, Jacobs C, Haag S, Wehrbein H. Apical root resorption during orthodontic treatment with aligners? A retrospective radiometric study. Head Face Med. 2013;14:21.
104. Barbagallo LJ, Jones AS, Petocz P, Darendeliler MA. Physical properties of root cementum: part 10. Comparison of the effects of invisible removable thermoplastic appliances with light and heavy orthodontic forces on premolar cementum. A microcomputed-tomography study. Am J Orthod Dentofacial Orthop. 2008;133(2):218–27.
105. Pandis N, Nasika M, Polychronopoulou A, Eliades T. External apical root resorption in patients treated with conventional and self-ligating brackets. Am J Orthod Dentofacial Orthop. 2008;134(5):646–51.
106. Leite V, Conti AC, Navarro R, Almeida M, Oltramari-Navarro P, Almeida R. Comparison of root resorption between self-ligating and conventional preadjusted brackets using cone beam computed tomography. Angle Orthod. 2012;82(6):1078–82.
107. Jacobs C, Gebhardt PF, Jacobs V, Hechtner M, Meila D, Wehrbein H. Root resorption, treatment time and extraction rate during orthodontic treatment with self-ligating and conventional brackets. Head Face Med. 2014;10(1):2.
108. Marques LS, Ramos-Jorge ML, Rey AC, Armond MC, Ruellas AC. Severe root resorption in orthodontic patients treated with the edgewise method: prevalence and predictive factors. Am J Orthod Dentofacial Orthop. 2010;137(3):384–8.
109. de Freitas MR, Beltrão RT, Janson G, Henriques JF, Chiqueto K. Evaluation of root resorption after open bite treatment with and without extractions. Am J Orthod Dentofacial Orthop. 2007;132(2):143.e15–22E.
110. Huang Y, Wang XX, Zhang J, Liu C, Huang Y, Wang XX, Zhang J, Liu C. Root shortening in patients treated with two-step and en masse space closure procedures with sliding mechanics. Angle Orthod. 2010;80(3):792–7.
111. Alzahawi K, Færøvig E, Brudvik P, Bøe O, Mavragani M. Root resorption after leveling with super-elastic and conventional steel arch wires: a prospective study. Prog Orthod. 2014; 15(1):35.
112. Weiland F. Constant versus dissipating forces in orthodontics: the effect on initial tooth movement and root resorption. Eur J Orthod. 2003;25:335–42.
113. Ballard DJ, Jones AS, Petocz P, Darendeliler MA. Physical properties of root cementum: part 11. Continuous vs intermittent controlled orthodontic forces on root resorption. A microcomputed-tomography study. Am J Orthod Dentofacial Orthop. 2009;136(1):8.e1–8; discussion 8–9.
114. Aras B, Cheng LL, Turk T, Elekdag-Turk S, Jones AS, Darendeliler MA. Physical properties of root cementum: part 23. Effects of 2 or 3 weekly reactivated continuous or intermittent orthodontic forces on root resorption and tooth movement: a microcomputed tomography study. Am J Orthod Dentofacial Orthop. 2012;14(2):e29–37.
115. Zahed Zahedani S, Oshagh M, Momeni Danaei S, Roeinpeikar S. A comparison of apical root resorption in incisors after fixed orthodontic treatment with standard edgewise and straight wire (MBT) method. J Dent. 2013;14(3):103–10.
116. Shoreibah EA, Salama AE, Attia MS, Abu-Seida SM. Corticotomy-facilitated orthodontics in adults using a further modified technique. J Int Acad Periodontol. 2012;14(4):97–104.
117. Janson G, Nakamura A, de Freitas MR, Henriques JF, Pinzan A. Apical root resorption comparison between Fränkel and eruption guidance appliances. Am J Orthod Dentofacial Orthop. 2007;131(6):729–35.

118. Tomizuka R, Kanetaka H, Shimizu Y, Suzuki A, Igarashi K, Mitani H. Effects of gradually increasing force generated by permanent rare earth magnets for orthodontic tooth movement. Angle Orthod. 2006;76(6):1004–9.
119. Brezniak N, Wasserstein A. Root resorption after orthodontic treatment: part 2. Am J Orthod Dentofacial Orthop. 1993;103(2):138–46.
120. Esteves T, Ramos AL, Pereira CM, Hidalgo MM. Orthodontic root resorption of endodontically treated teeth. J Endod. 2007;33(2):119–22.
121. Haug SR, Brudvik P, Fristad I, Heyeraas KJ. Sympathectomy causes increased root resorption after orthodontic tooth movement in rats: immunohistochemical study. Cell Tissue Res. 2003;313(2):167–75.
122. Fonseca PD, de Lima FM, Higashi DT, Koyama DF, Toginho Filho Dde O, Dias IF, Ramos Sde P. Effects of light emitting diode (LED) therapy at 940 nm on inflammatory root resorption in rats. Lasers Med Sci. 2013;28(1):49–55.
123. Liu Z, Xu J, L E, Wang D. Ultrasound enhances the healing of orthodontically induced root resorption in rats. Angle Orthod. 2012;82(1):48–55.
124. El-Bialy T, El-Shamy I, Graber TM. Repair of orthodontically induced root resorption by ultrasound in humans. Am J Orthod Dentofacial Orthop. 2004;123(2):186–93.
125. Marshall JA. A comparison of resorption of roots of deciduous teeth with the absorption of roots of the permanent teeth occurring as a result of infection. Int J Orthod. 1929;15:417.
126. Brcks H. Root resorption and their relation to pathologic bone formation. Int J Orthod. 1939;22:445–82.
127. Hedgecoe A. Politics of personalised medicine: pharmacogenetics in the clinic. s.l. Cambridge: Cambridge University Press; 2004.
128. Abbas AK. In: Abbas AK, Lichtman AH, Pillai S. editors. Cellular and molecular immunology. Properties and Overview of Immune system. Philadelphia: Saunders; 2011.
129. Al-Qawasmi RA, Hartsfield Jr JK, Everett ET, Flury L, Liu L, Foroud TM, Macri JV, Roberts WE. Genetic predisposition of external apical root resorption in orthodontic patients: linkage of chromosome 18 marker. J Dent Res. 2005;82(5):356–60.
130. Luciani F, Bull RA, Lloyd AR. Next generation deep sequencing and vaccine design: today and tomorrow. Trends Biotechnol. 2012;30(9):443–52.
131. Geisler M, Sornette D, Woodard R. Exuberant innovation: the Human Genome Project. 10–12, Apr 2010, Swiss Finance Institute Research Paper No 10–12; 2010.
132. MIT. The rise and fall of the Human Genome Project. Technology review; 2010.
133. Venter CJ, Adams MG, Meyers EW, et al. The sequence of the human genome. Science. 2001;291:1304–51.
134. Tinoco I Jr., et al. Report on the Human Genome Initiative. US Department of Energy; 1987. Human Genome Project Information.
135. Baumert U, Golan I, Becker B, Hrala BP, Redlich M, Roos HA, Palmon A, Reichenberg E, Müssig D. Pressure simulation of orthodontic force in osteoblasts: a pilot study. Orthod Craniofac Res. 2004;7(1):3–9.
136. Ben-Zvi I, Brandt N, Berkun Y, Lidar M, Livneh A. The relative contribution of environmental and genetic factors to phenotypic variation in familial Mediterranean fever (FMF). Gene. 2012;491:260–3.
137. Latour B. Science in action: how to follow scientists and engineers through society. s. l. Cambridge: Harvard University Press; 1987.
138. Reichenberg E, Redlich M, Cancemi P, Zaks B, Pitaru S, Fontana S, Pucci-Minafra I, Palmon A. Proteomic analysis of protein components in periodontal ligament fibroblasts. J Periodontol. 2005;76(10):1645–53.
139. Masella RS, Meister M. Current concepts on the orthodontic tooth movement. Am J Orthod Dentofacial Orthop. 2006;129(4):458–68.
140. Harris EF. Root resorption during orthodontic therapy. Semin Orthod. 2000;6:183–94.
141. Harris EF, Kineret SE, Tolley EA. A heritable component for external apical root resorption in patients treated orthodontically. Am J Orthod Dentofacial Orthop. 1997;111(3):301–9.

142. Hartsfield JK Jr. In: Vanarsdall RL Jr, Vig KWJ, Graber LW, editors. Orthodontics current principles and techniques. 5th ed. s. l. Mosby; 2012. p. 209–45. Genetics and Orthodontics.
143. Deane S, Jones AS, Petocz P, Darendeliler MA. Physical properties of root cementum: part 12. The incidence of physiologic root resorption on unerupted third molars and its comparison with orthodontically treated premolars: a microcomputed-tomography study. Am J Orthod Dentofacial Orthop. 2009;136(2):148.e1–9; discussion 148–9.
144. Srivicharnkul P, Kharbanda OP, Swain MV, Petocz P, Darendeliler MA. Physical properties of root cementum: part 3. Hardness and elastic modulus after application of light and heavy forces. Am J Orthod Dentofacial Orthop. 2005;127(2):168–76.
145. Merckmanuals. www.merckmanuals.com. [Online] [Cited: 27 Dec 2014]. http://www.merckmanuals.com/professional/critical_care_medicine/shock_and_fluid_resuscitation/shock.html.
146. PM B. Studies in mammalian dentition. Differentiation of canine. Proc Zool Soc Lond (Series B). 1939;109:1.
147. Graber LW. Congenital absence of teeth: a review with emphasis on inheritance pattern. J Am Dent Assoc. 1978;96:266–75.
148. Mirabella AD, Artun J. Prevalence and severity of apical root resorption of maxillary anterior teeth in adult orthodontic patients. Eur J Orthod. 1995;17:93–9.
149. Smith RJ, Burstone CJ. Mechanics of tooth movement. Am J Orthod. 1984;85(4):294–307.
150. Braun E. Genes? Certainly not all in life. Odyssey: Published in Hebrew; 2009
151. Levander E, Bajka R, Malmgren O. Early radiographic diagnosis of apical root resorption during orthodontic treatment: a study of maxillary incisors. Eur J Orthod. 1998;20(1):57–63.
152. Levander E, Malmgren O. Long-term follow-up of maxillary incisors with severe apical root resorption. Eur J Orthod. 2000;22:85–92.
153. Grünheid T, Kolbeck Schieck JR, Pliska BT, Ahmad M, Larson BE. Dosimetry of a cone-beam computed tomography machine compared with a digital x-ray machine in orthodontic imaging. Am J Orthod Dentofacial Orthop. 2012;141(4):436–43.
154. Field C, Ichim I, Swain MV, Chan E, Darendeliler MA, Li W, Li Q. Mechanical responses to orthodontic loading: a 3-dimensional finite element multi-tooth model. Am J Orthod Dentofacial Orthop. 2009;135(2):174–81.
155. Roberts WE, Turley PK, Brezniak N, Fielder PJ. Implants: bone physiology and metabolism. CDA J. 1987;15(10):54–64.
156. Gillespie MT. Impact of cytokines and T lymphocytes upon osteoclast differentiation and function. Arthritis Res Ther. 2007;9:103.
157. Takayanagi H. Osteoimmunology: shared mechanisms and crosstalk between the immune and bone systems. Nature Reviews. Immunology. 2007;7:292–304.
158. Wheeler TT, Stroup SE. Traumatic root resorption in dentine immunized mice. Am J Orthod Dentofacial Orthop. 1993;104:352–7.
159. Hidalgo MM, Itano EN, Consolaro A. Humoral immune response of patients with dental trauma and consequent replacement resorption. Dent Traumatol. 2005;21(4):218–21.
160. Brezniak N, Goren S, Zoizner R, Dinbar A, Arad A, Wasserstein A, Heller M. A comparison of three methods to accurately measure root length. Angle Orthod. 2004;74(6):786–91.
161. Brezniak N, Goren S, Zoizner R, Dinbar A, Arad A, Wasserstein A, Heller M. The use of an individual jig in measuring tooth length changes. Angle Orthod. 2004;74:780–5.
162. Brin I, Tulloch JF, Koroluk L, Philips C. External apical root resorption in class II malocclusion: a retrospective review of 1- versus 2-phase treatment. Am J Orthod Dentofacial Orthop. 2003;124(2):151–6.
163. Karadeniz EI, Gonzales C, Turk T, Isci D, Sahin-Saglam AM, Alkis H, Elekdag-Turk S, Darendeliler MA. Effect of fluoride on root resorption following heavy and light orthodontic force application for 4 weeks and 12 weeks of retention. Angle Orthod. 2013;83(3):418–24.
164. Inubushi T, Tanaka E, Rego EB, Ohtani J, Kawazoe A, Tanne K, Miyauchi M, Takata T. Ultrasound stimulation attenuates resorption of tooth root induced by experimental force application. Bone. 2013;53(2):497–506.

Genetic Implications in Orthodontic Tooth Movement

5

James K. Hartsfield Jr. and Lorri Ann Morford

Abstract

In orthodontics there is an interest in understanding how orthodontic tooth movement (OTM) may be modified with the use of differential anchorage and decreasing treatment time(s). While the focus of these efforts has been on how various procedures or devices affect OTM (i.e., typically increase OTM), there has been little discussion of how the patient's genetic background may influence variation in OTM. In this chapter, the clinician will be introduced to basic concepts of clinical genetics to gain insight into various genetic factors that influence bone modeling/remodeling and OTM. We describe how the genetic factors in these important pathways may also influence external apical root resorption (EARR) concurrent with OTM. At the end of the chapter, known genetic factors in two conditions that could secondarily affect OTM as they increase treatment complexity (dental primary failure of eruption and dental agenesis) are reviewed, and a select group of syndromes and other genetic conditions that may affect OTM in patients are also summarized.

5.1 Introduction to Types of Genetic Factors

Genetic factors influence numerous biological processes including orthodontic tooth movement (OTM), external apical root resorption that can be seen on standard radiographs (EARR), and problems with tooth formation and/or eruption. Therefore,

J.K. Hartsfield Jr., DMD, MS, MMSC, PhD, FACMG, CDABO (✉) • L.A. Morford PhD
Center for the Biologic Basis of Oral/Systemic Diseases, Hereditary Genetics/Genomics Core, Department of Oral Health Science, University of Kentucky College of Dentistry, 1095 Veterans Administration Drive, 414 Health Science Research Building (HSRB), Lexington, KY 40536-0305, USA
e-mail: James.Hartsfield@uky.edu; lorri.morford@uky.edu

B. Shroff (ed.), *Biology of Orthodontic Tooth Movement*,
DOI 10.1007/978-3-319-26609-1_5

when a clinician has a good understanding of the genetic factors that influence OTM and some of the genetically influenced problems associated with OTM, treatment outcomes can be improved for many of their patients. A *genetic factor* can be defined as a gene or a specific gene variation that has an effect on some characteristic(s) of an individual or their offspring, where a *gene* is the smallest unit of inherited information. Inherited and newly introduced (sporadic) gene variations may be defined simply as a single nucleotide change at a specific location in the DNA code (i.e., a polymorphism), or they could consist of deletions, insertions, amplifications/duplications, inversions, and/or transposition of larger portions of the DNA code.

Genetic factors can be studied from different perspectives including (1) determining how many unique genetic factors are needed to influence a biological process such that there is a measurable effect or discernible difference in the phenotype (the observable properties, measurable features, and physical characteristics of the patient) and (2) determining the nature of how each factor influences the phenotype (i.e., does it primarily alter the structure and/or function of the protein made from the genetic code? Does it alter how much of the protein is? Or both?). By studying these different perspectives, scientists and clinicians help to relate a patient's genetic background (called the *genome* in total or *genotype* when referring to a specific genetic variation) to the phenotype of the patient [12]. A *phenotype* is generated by the summation and interaction of the effects arising over a period of time from an individual's genotype and the effects of environment in which the individual develops within. A *trait* is one particular aspect or characteristic of the phenotype.

5.1.1 How Many Genetic Factors Are Necessary to Have an Effect or Make a Discernible Difference?

If a trait arises due to the effect of a single gene being expressed or due to a unique variation in that gene, then the trait is said to have Mendelian (i.e., monogenic; mono = "*one*", genic = "*gene*") inheritance. Use of the terms autosomal dominant, autosomal recessive, or X-linked modes of inheritance can further describe the specific subtypes of Mendelian inheritance. For example, an autosomal dominant (AD) monogenic pattern of inheritance occurs when only one copy of the trait-causing genetic factor is needed to inherit the trait. Theoretically, each child of an individual with an AD trait has a 50 % chance of inheriting the same AD trait. The inheritance of an AD trait, however, is not always so simple or straightforward.

When a family tree (called a pedigree in genetics) is drawn specifically indicating the family members who have and do not have the trait, it may be discovered that the appearance of the trait "skips a generation." In clinical genetic terms, the trait is then said to be *non-penetrant* (e.g., a person does not show the trait themselves, yet they inherited the same genetic variation that runs in the family and is associated with the trait and can pass it on to their children who may show the trait). In addition, among family members who show the trait, the trait may not be apparent to the same extent or severity from one individual to the next. In clinical genetic terms, this phenomenon is referred to as *variable expressivity*. How is this possible for a trait that is said to be AD? These variations in the appearance of an AD trait occur because proteins and/or RNA products from other genes, together with environmental factor effects, can cause differences in how the trait is expressed or if the trait will be expressed at all in a particular individual (even though the individual has a variation in a single gene that is usually associated with the trait).

Simply stated, an AD monogenic trait is caused by a single gene, but the actual outward appearance of the trait is determined by the combined effect of other inherited factors that modify the extent or severity of the appearance of the trait. For example, the occurrences of dental agenesis (hypodontia/oligodontia) are AD in most of the reported families, with observed variations in the type and/or number of teeth that are affected and with a tendency for other teeth that are present in the dentition to be small. In contrast to an AD pattern of inheritance, an autosomal recessive mode of inheritance of a trait describes the case when two copies of the trait-causing genetic factor are needed to show the trait; and X-linked modes of inheritance specifically involve the inheritance of trait-causing genetic factors from the X-chromosome.

However, most clinically observed traits do not display a monogenic inheritance. They instead may tend to "run in families," but do not exhibit a pattern of inheritance that is as extensive or as well defined as would be expected with Mendelian (monogenic) traits. These conditions are referred to as *complex or common traits*, reflecting their complex etiological interaction between multiple and environmental factors, as well as their greater incidence/more common occurrence when compared to monogenic traits. Because so many genetic and environmental factors come into play with a complex trait, this type of trait is usually assessed using a continuous or quantitative measurement, not a discrete "yes" or "no" occurrence. Thus, one may expect that when compared to monogenic traits, complex traits will be more amenable to change (or a greater change) following environmental/treatment modification (e.g., OTM).

5.1.2 What Is the Nature of Each Genetic Factor Involved in Forming a Specific Trait?

The process of utilizing the instructions contained within our DNA code is called *gene expression*. During this process, the information contained within a gene can be copied into an RNA template to be used to synthesize a protein product that was encoded by the DNA instructions. Some DNA codes don't make protein directly, but contain the needed instructions to produce different types of regulatory RNA molecules (e.g., microRNAs, long non-coding RNAs, etc.). These regulatory molecules usually help to define where and how much of a specific protein should be made by specifically targeting the protein-encoding RNA template for destruction when it is no longer needed.

When we study the effect of genetic variation on gene expression, two main mechanisms in our bodies can influence the effectiveness and/or amount of a protein being made and, in doing so, can influence our observable and/or measurable traits. With the first mechanism, an inherited or sporadic variation in the DNA code of a gene results in a change in the amino acid sequence of the protein being produced. Extreme and/or strategic amino acid sequence changes could (a) result in an altered function of the protein (i.e., making it either inactive or hyperactive), (b) introduce a *STOP* code into the protein resulting in the formation of a truncated protein, complete absence of the protein, and/or a signal to quickly destroy the protein, or (c) alter how a protein is localized within the cell (i.e., no longer sending it to its specific location of action). With the second mechanism, a genetic variation may influence how much of the protein is made. Genetic variations in the regulatory region in front of a gene code (called promoter regions) may influence when or for how long a gene is "turned on" (i.e., expressed to form a protein or regulatory RNA). Similarly, genetic variations found within the DNA code of the gene that cause the RNA and protein-producing machinery to stop or pause can also influence how much protein is synthesized. As an analogy to understand these two concepts, think of water coming out of a garden hose. In the first instance, water (protein) is coming out of the hose (is being made from the gene), but the water may be partly or completely adulterated by contamination (due to a detrimental variation or mutation in the gene). In the second instance, good water is coming out of the hose, but there is less or more of it than is needed. Of course, both could happen at the same time with water hoses, as well as with genes and their associated proteins.

There are many genetic and environmental factors that will turn genes "*off*" and/or "*on*" or that can change the rate of the proteins being made. With orthodontic force, the stress of the root against the periodontal ligament (PDL) and alveolar bone will cause changes in the gene expression and corresponding protein production for numerous genes, ultimately resulting in the changes in the shape of the socket ("modeling" as discussed later) so the tooth will move. In the remainder of the chapter, specific genetic variations that can affect OTM will be reviewed, as well as their possible relationship with EARR. In addition, genetic factors affecting primary failure of eruption, agenic teeth, and selected syndromes that may be associated with an effect on, or a concern about, OTM will be reviewed.

5.2 Genetic Factors Associated with Variation(s) in OTM

Knowledge of the cellular and molecular processes that are regulated in response to placing physical stress on the tissues supporting and surrounding a tooth help us to understand the mechanism(s) by which OTM occurs. Understanding these cellular and molecular processes can also help suggest what genes should be studied for genetic variation that might contribute to the differences observed with OTM clinically. Many animal studies and a limited number of human studies have attempted to measure variations in the gene expression of numerous proteins following the placement of an orthodontic force on a tooth. These studies have been instrumental in identifying specific cytokines, chemokines, hormones, growth factors, enzymes, neuropeptides, and ligands that influence OTM.

Most of these studies, however, have used the term "*remodeling*" to indicate a change in the gross morphology of the boney socket observed with OTM, echoing the same usage to describe and understand the surface sculpting and drift mechanisms of facial growth and development [42]. While orthodontic investigators have tended to embrace the term "remodeling" to describe this bone surface change, mineralized tissue biologists have used the term "*modeling*" for this activity, reserving the term "*remodeling*" to describe internal bone turnover mechanisms that do not change the shape of the bone. Unfortunately, this difference in term usage by many in orthodontic research has created confusion in a variety of scientific circles and has acted as a barrier to the exchange of information with other biomedical disciplines [139, 140]. For the sake of clarity, we will use the terms "modeling" and "remodeling" in this chapter as defined by mineralized tissue biologists.

Multiple molecular pathways that influence OTM have been identified to date [118], as well as many pathways that influence processes associated with OTM, such as root resorption on the histological level as typically seen in extracted teeth (RR) and EARR as typically seen on standard radiographs [58]. Two of the pathways influencing both OTM and RR/EARR include the ATP/P2XR7/IL-1B inflammatory signaling pathway and the RANKL/RANK/OPG bone modeling/remodeling pathway, both which are illustrated in Fig. 5.1. Yet, even with this knowledge of key pathways influencing OTM, few studies have focused on determining how actual variations in nonsyndromic genetic factors correlate with the actual clinical outcomes observed during OTM in humans.

The best examples are the investigations by Iwasaki, Nickel, and colleagues [74, 75, 77]. This group applied a simple model based on disease processes to study the multiple factors that affect the normal physiological phenomenon of OTM (Fig. 5.2). In this model system, the phenotype (speed of OTM) is the result of environmental and genetic factors and their interaction. Unless the patient has a condition that overwhelms all other factors like some of those mentioned later in Sect. 5.5, the etiology of both OTM and RR/EARR is likely to be complex, i.e., the result of many factors, each of which may only account for a relatively small portion of the clinical variability seen.

Iwasaki et al. also proposed a diagrammatic structure for future research on the effect of various conditions and the variations (polymorphisms) for specific genes (Fig. 5.3). This would require both a precise and accurate measure of tooth movement (ideally bodily with stress along the length of the PDL evenly distributed as much as possible) under defined forces, along with comprehensive analysis of genetic variation, the scale of which has to date not been done. However, this has been done choosing genetic variation markers based on part of the ATP/P2RX7/IL-1B pathway, the genes for IL-1β and another related cytokine IL-1α (*IL1B* and *IL1A*, respectively), and the gene (*IL1RN*) for another molecular (IL-1 receptor antagonist, IL-RA) that helps to regulate their biological activity.

Interleukin-1 (IL-1) is a polypeptide primarily produced by cells of mononuclear phagocyte lineage that generally promotes proinflammatory responses [41]. One of the types of cells affected is osteoblasts, resulting in a potent stimulation of bone resorption in vitro and in vivo by inducing osteoblasts to promote the activity of

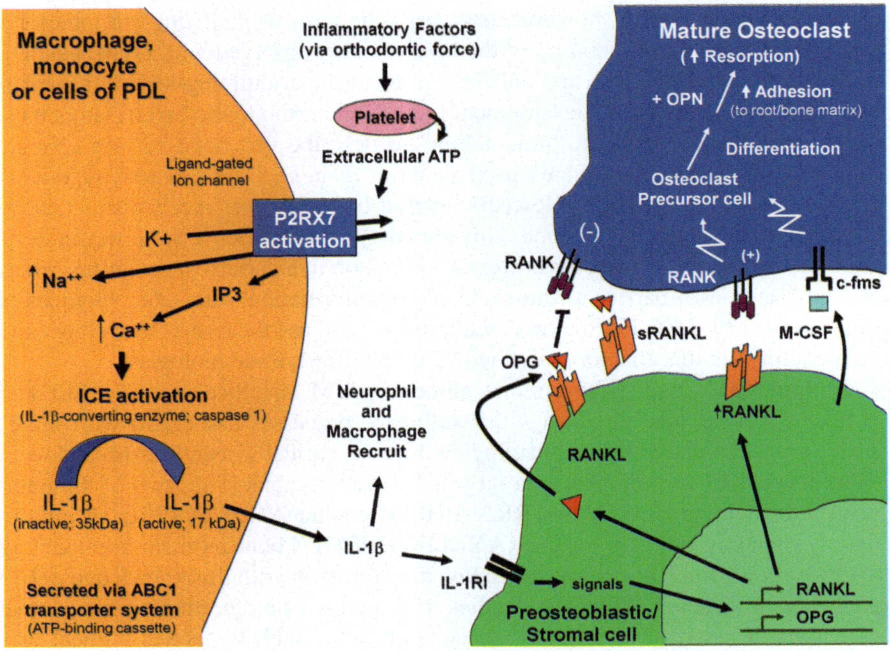

Fig. 5.1 As orthodontic force is placed on the teeth and the neighboring periodontal ligament (PDL) is compressed, the immune system responds at the site to relieve the tissue stress. As part of the stress response, ATP is released from platelets and can bind to the P2RX7 membrane channel protein located on the surface of immune cells and/or cells of the PDL. Upon binding ATP, the P2RX7 ion channel is opened, allowing the exchange of intracellular potassium (*K+*) and extracellular sodium (*Na*++), along with triggering the elevation of calcium (*Ca*++) from intracellular stores. Elevation of intracellular Ca++ will activate caspase-1 (also termed IL-1β converting enzyme or ICE) which is located in inflammasome complexes with the cell (not depicted). Caspase-1 cleaves the pro-IL-1β molecule, releasing active mature IL-1β for biological function. IL-1β can recruit other inflammatory cells to the site of tissue damage, and it can bind to its receptor on the surface of pro-osteoblastic cells in order to signal the activation of such genes as RANKL and OPG. When RANKL protein is synthesized and expressed on the surface of the osteoblastic cells, in concert with the production of M-CSF and its binding to the c-fms receptor on the surface of pre-osteoclastic cells, the osteoclast precursor cells are signaled to mature into functional osteoclasts. OPG and soluble RANKL (*sRANKL*) can act to dampen the maturation signal to pro-osteoclast cells by interfering with RANKL:RANK interactions. The action of both osteoblasts and osteoclasts is needed to resolve the tissue stresses within the PDL from orthodontic force application

osteoclasts [92]. Interleukin-1 comes in α- and β-forms, each coded by a separate gene. Of these two forms, IL-1β is the most potent for bone resorption and inhibition of bone formation [151]. OTM requires a balance between IL-1β and IL-1RA synthesis for the bone modeling and remodeling processes involved.

Variation in the ratio of IL-1β-1RA protein found in gingival crevicular fluid (GCF) has accounted for 52–72 % of the inter-individual differences observed in the rate of OTM, and this finding correlated with the *IL1B* (rs1143634, also termed +3954) and *ILRN* ($VNTR_{86bp}$) genetic variations (alleles) inherited by each subject examined [73, 74, 76]. Previous studies have shown that these genetic variations can influence the

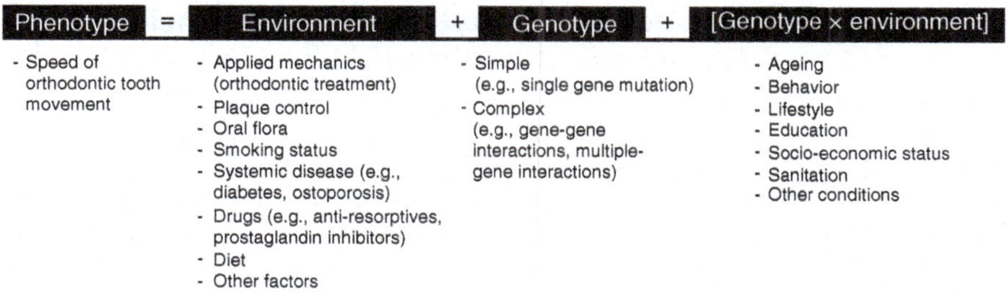

Fig. 5.2 Model of factors affecting phenotype (Reproduced with permission from *Semin Orthod.* 2008;14:135–45. © *2008 Elsevier Inc*)

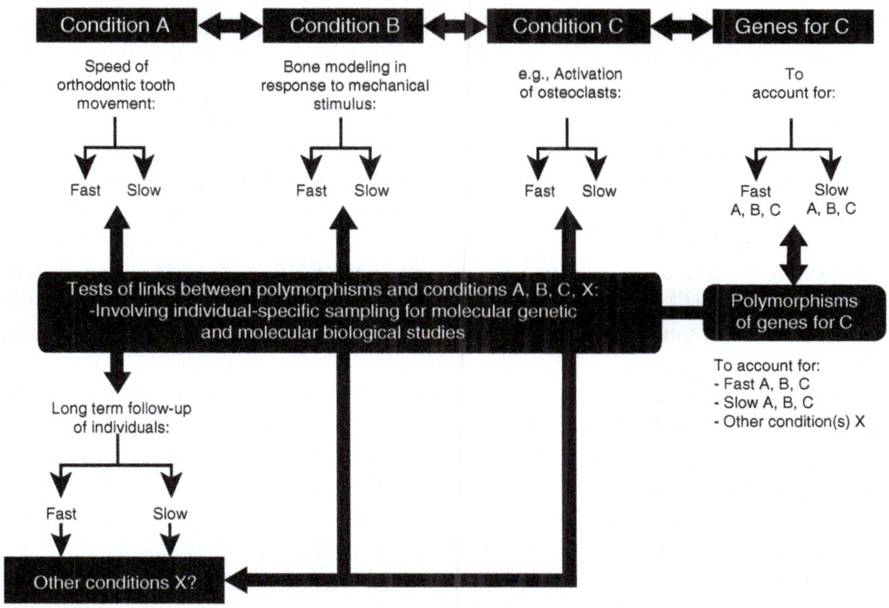

Fig. 5.3 Proposed approach to orthodontic tooth movement/polymorphism association (Reproduced with permission from *Semin Orthod.* 2008;14:135–45. © *2008 Elsevier Inc*)

amount of IL1B and ILRN protein that is produced/secreted. For example, the of this specific *IL1B* genetic variation called the A1 allele in one copy, and particularly two copies, has been associated with an increase in IL-1β secretion two- and four-fold respectively [131]. Having the specific variation in the *ILRN* gene with at least one copy of allele 2 (A2+) is associated with an increase in secretion of the ILRA molecule, which would decrease the number of open receptor binding sites for IL1β and therefore decrease its effect [35, 65]. The velocity of maxillary canine OTM retraction was greater with 26 kPa of force than with 13 or 52 kPa, with a high IL-1β/IL1-RA protein ratio in the GCF, when the individual inherited two *IL1B* A1 alleles, and in the absence of any A2+ alleles for the *ILRN* gene. Analysis of a DNA marker in the *IL1A* gene was not associated with variation in OTM [76].

5.3 Relationships Between Genetic Factors Influencing External Apical Root Resorption (EARR) and Variations in OTM

EARR can occur in the absence of orthodontia, particularly in individuals with missing teeth, increased periodontal probing depths, reduced crestal bone heights, bruxism, chronic nail-biting, and anterior open bites with concomitant tongue thrust [54, 56]. EARR is also increased as a pathologic consequence of orthodontic mechanical loading in some patients [21, 22]. The amount of orthodontic movement is positively associated with the resulting extent of EARR [39, 126, 147]. Orthodontic tooth movement, or "biomechanics," has been found to account for approximately one-tenth to one-third of the total variation in EARR [14, 64, 95]. Owman-Moll and coworkers [125] showed that individual variation overshadowed the force magnitude and the force type in defining the susceptibility to histological root resorption associated with orthodontic force. Individual variations were considerable regarding both extension and depth of RR within individuals, and these were not correlated to the magnitude of tooth movement achieved [90].

As has been observed with velocity of OTM, there is individual variation in EARR associated with orthodontic treatment, indicating an individual predisposition and multifactorial (complex) etiology [55, 104, 105, 119, 137, 142]. Genetic variations with the *IL-1* gene have been investigated and appear to be associated with EARR (Fig. 5.4). The *IL1B* A2 allele (+3954, single nucleotide polymorphism (SNP) rs1143634) associated with decreased IL-1β secretion has been associated with an increased incidence of EARR in orthodontic patients in some studies [3, 13, 67] and has also been shown to associate with slower OTM [76]. Other studies, however, have failed to find an association between the IL1B A2 allele and EARR in orthodontic patients. For example, in a population of German orthodontic patients a polymorphism in the *IL1A* gene promoter (-889) was associated with EARR, while an *IL1B* +3954 genetic marker was not [51]. Moreover, no association was apparent between EARR and *IL-1β* SNP +3954 in a recent meta-analysis [168].

This is not be surprising since as only one factor in the complex process of EARR, variation in *IL1B* had only accounted for 15 % of the variation in EARR in the original study [3], leaving a lot (85 %) of variation to be accounted for my other genetic and non-genetic factors. From 2003 to 2015 there have been several genetic studies published looking at various genetic markers in genes that were postulated to potentially affect EARR in orthodontic patients (Fig. 5.5). They have largely investigated DNA markers in genes of either the ATP/P2RX7/IL1B or the RANKL/RANK/OPG pathways. Gene polymorphisms have also been studied for association with EARR including within the TNFα gene, which encodes a cytokine that is increased during OTM; the tissue nonspecific alkaline phosphatase genes (*TNSALP*, also known as alkaline phosphatase liver/bone/kidney or ALPL), which is mentioned in Section 5.5 for its role in hypophosphatasia; the osteopontin gene (*OPN*) which can influence osteoblast attachment to the surface to be demineralized; and the gene for the vitamin D receptor (*VDR*).

More recently studies are including multiple treatment and genetic factors in models to explain the occurrence of EARR concurrent with orthodontia. For example, in

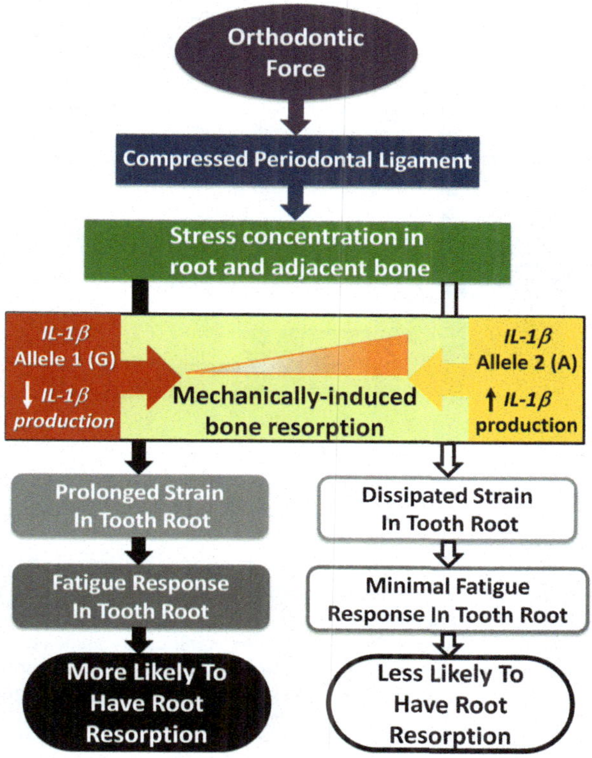

Fig. 5.4 Proposed model for pathway through which *IL-1B* genotype modulates the extent of root resorption experienced during orthodontic tooth movement. This model suggests that low IL-1 production in case of allele 1 (*G*) results in relatively less catabolic bone modeling in cortical bone interface of periodontal ligament (PDL) because of decreased number of osteoclasts associated with lower levels of this cytokine. Inhibition of bone resorption in direction of tooth movement results in maintaining prolonged dynamic loading of tooth root adjacent to compressed PDL, resulting in more root resorption because of fatigue failure of root. In case of high IL-1 production associated with allele 2 (*A*), compressed PDL space is restored by resorption of bone interface of PDL, resulting in only mild root resorption that is controlled by cementum-healing mechanism. This is 1 model for how these various factors might be implicated in clinical expression of root resorption (Reproduced with permission from *Am J Orthod Dentofacial Orthop*. 2003;123:242–52)

one study 30 % of the EARR variability was explained by variation in treatment duration, the use of a Hyrax appliance, premolar extractions, sex, and the *P2RX7* gene rs1718119 SNP, while age, overjet, tongue thrust, skeletal class II, and other genetic polymorphisms made only minor contributions [129]. Similarly, a second study examined the relative influence of multiple parameters on the occurrence of EARR including treatment duration, extraction of maxillary premolars, and numerous cephalometric measurements (pretreatment, post-treatment, and overall change in values), as well as genotypes for multiple DNA polymorphisms. This study found that a longer length of treatment, missing or extracted maxillary premolars, changes in

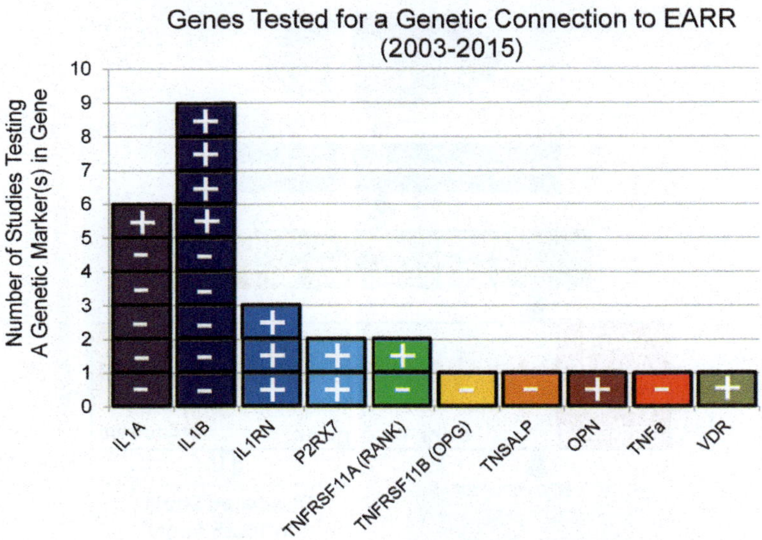

Fig. 5.5 Several genetic variants have been investigated in association with the presence of external apical root resorption (EARR) concurrent with orthodontia, in a number of populations, and using various methods of EARR assessment. Each plus sign in a box above a gene indicates that at least one genetic marker in that gene was found to be significantly associated with EARR in a published study, while a minus sign indicates that markers in that gene were not significantly associated with EARR. Markers in some of the genes have been evaluated in more than one study (Refs. [3, 4, 45, 51, 68–72, 96, 146])

cephalomentric FMA and Ur-pvt, and specific polymorphisms in the *P2RX7*, *IL-1β*, and *CASP-1/ICE* genes together explained 25 % of the total variation associated with EARR concurrent with orthodontia in the sample tested [146].

These studies are interesting in that they emphasize the possible effect of longer treatment times on EARR concurrent with orthodontia and support the involvement of the ATP/P2RX7/IL1B pathway since the P2RX7 protein is an upstream regulator of the activation of IL-1β that was a focus of initial studies [58]. In an inbred mouse model with the mouse version of the *P2RX7* gene knocked out showed an increase in histological root resorption with orthodontic force [161], as did a previous inbred mouse model with the mouse version of the *IL1B* gene knocked out [5].

While a genetic connection between velocity of OTM and an inverse likelihood of EARR has been proposed and tentatively supported, much more needs to be done. Recently there has been much interest in various means to safely increase the velocity of OTM to shorten treatment time without an increase in EARR or other negative sequelae. Unfortunately, describing or measuring the underlying genetics that could influence part of the overall phenotypic variation seen clinically with OTM and changes with adjunctive therapy or devices designed to increase or accelerate OTM, is often is missing in OTM research studies, as well as in investigations examining the effects of treatment modalities on growth. Ultimately evidence-based orthodontic practice guidelines that do not take into account genetic differences may be lacking a substantial aspect of what influences the clinical outcome [59].

5.4 Genetic Factors in Dental Primary Failure of Eruption and Agenesis

Primary failure of eruption and dental agenesis (hypodontia and oligodontia) are conditions that often have a strong or dominant genetic etiology and secondary affect OTM as they increase treatment complexity. Some genetic factors that influence the occurrence of these traits are described below.

5.4.1 Primary Failure of Eruption (Nonsyndromic)

In contrast to failure of teeth to erupt associated with mechanical failure of eruption (e.g., cysts, gingival fibromatosis, adjacent teeth) or with syndromes like cleidocranial dysplasia, primary failure of eruption (PFE) is a disorder in which a tooth will not erupt, typically along with all teeth distal to the most mesial involved tooth, *nor* will the affected teeth respond to orthodontic force. The familial occurrence of this phenotype in approximately one-quarter of all cases facilitated the investigation and discovery of genetic variations within the *PTHR1* gene associated with the disorder [38, 133]. In addition to diagnosis of individuals who are likely to develop or have PFE, a better understanding of its etiology could result in a molecular treatment for PFE, as well as the manipulation of selective tooth eruption rates to enhance treatment protocols on an individual basis [152, 166].

The clinical impact of PFE is frequently very severe, with impairment of alveolar bone growth in the affected areas. The affected teeth appear at the base of a large vertical bony defect and often present dilacerations, resulting in a severe lateral open bite. Unfortunately the affected teeth typically become ankylosed as soon as orthodontic force is applied [134, 135]. It is not clear why highly variable clinical expressivity is observed in PFE, with some persons affected bilaterally and others affected unilaterally in the same family. There is also no apparent explanation for why the posterior dentition is preferentially affected. To date, there are only a few anecdotal cases of successful extrusion of teeth affected with PFE. Thus, any attempt at early orthodontic intervention involving affected teeth for these patients has been said to be futile [47]. The best treatment for an accurately established early diagnosis of PFE is initially no treatment of the affected teeth, reserving the multidisciplinary options for affected patients for a later time after the completion of growth [47].

5.4.2 Dental Agenesis

Dental development is a complex process that requires over 300 different genes working together to provide the instructions needed to form a full complement of teeth (http://bite-it.helsinki.fi). This intricate process is not only regulated spatially within three dimensions but in a time-dependent manner [110]. Genetic mutations or variations in one or more of the required developmental genes can alter the normal process of tooth formation and may result in dental anomalies such as agenesis, small teeth, and/or peg-shaped teeth. In addition to affecting a patients' appearance, the number and type of naturally missing (agenic) teeth can contribute to problems with occlusion, alveolar bone growth and maintenance, periodontal health, mastication, and speech. The increased need for space closure and moving of shifted teeth can increase orthodontic treatment times and expense; hence early diagnosis can aid in proper treatment planning.

Dental agenesis is defined as the lack of formation of one or more teeth and can occur in the primary and/or the permanent dentition(s). The term "hypodontia" is used to describe the trait where 1–5 teeth fail to develop within the primary dentition or permanent dentition (excluding 3rd molars). In contrast, oligodontia is the lack of development of 6 or more teeth in the primary dentition or permanent dentition (excluding 3rd molars); and anodontia is a rare condition in which the entire permanent dentition fails to form. Agenic teeth may occur without the manifestation of other phenotypic features (i.e., nonsyndromic agenesis) or as one of many features associated with a syndrome.

Genetic, epigenetic, and environmental factors can all influence the occurrence of dental agenesis [23]. Individuals from families with a history of incisor/premolar agenesis will show an increased occurrence of other dental anomalies such as small or peg-shaped maxillary lateral incisors, displaced canines, taurodontism, and rotated premolars [6]. The mesial-distal crowns of all tooth types in hypodontia patients are smaller in size when compared to teeth from individuals forming a full complement of teeth such that the more severe the hypodontia, the smaller the size of the formed teeth [24].

Cusp pattern on the developed teeth in individuals with hypodontia is also altered compared to controls [84]. In addition, relatives within affected families who do not have agenesis may manifest teeth smaller in size than normal [24]. In stark contrast, patients with supernumerary teeth can present with larger than normal mesial-distal widths for their permanent maxillary incisors and canines than controls. Together, these observations suggest that there is a multigene (polygenic) influence on tooth size and patterning; and the occurrence of the variable pattern of hypodontia in some families is dependent on the combined input of multiple factors. Some known environmental influences for agenic teeth include inadequate nutrition, trauma, infection of the developing tooth bud, exposure to radiation, chemotherapy, drug exposure, and systemic diseases (i.e., rickets, syphilis, and rubella) [7]. Underlying mechanisms for many forms of dental agenesis are largely unknown.

5.4.3 Dental Agenesis in the Permanent Dentition

The worldwide prevalence of 3rd-molar agenesis is relative high at ~22.63 % (range 5.32–56 %), with African populations showing the lowest occurrence (mean = 5.74 %) and Asian populations showing the highest occurrence (mean = 29.71 %) [29]. Individuals with 3rd-molar agenesis are most likely to be missing 1–2 third molars and represent 8.44 and 7.79 % of the entire world population, respectively. The lack of 3 or 4 third molars is seen 2.53–3.42 % of people worldwide, accordingly [29]. Due to its relatively common occurrence, 3rd-molar agenesis is usually described separately from the agenesis of other tooth types within the human dentition.

The first genome-wide association study (GWAS) of 3rd-molar agenesis was conducted in 2013 with an Asian population [52]. This study identified three SNPs within the genome with a $p < 1 \times 10^{-5}$, with the most significant SNP, rs1469622, located within the thrombospondin type I domain-containing protein 7B (*THSD7B*) gene ($p = 7.5 \times 10^{-6}$; odds ratio 1.88, 95 % CI 1.43–2.47) [52]. While not confirmed in the Asian study, other genes have been implicated in 3rd-molar agenesis including the paired box 9 (*PAX9*), axis inhibitor 2 (*AXIN2*), and muscle segment homeobox 1 (*MSX1*) genes [91, 154, 160].

The prevalence of non-3rd-molar dental agenesis in the permanent dentition varies by ethnic group [85]. Worldwide prevalence ranges from 0.3 to 25.7 % [2]. However, studying orthodontic patients versus individuals within the general population can lead to broad variation in the numbers, possibly due to a bias in referral for orthodontic treatment in patients with dental agenesis [85]. The prevalence of hypodontia in the USA ranges from 1.6 to 8.8 %. Oligodontia is seen in ~0.3 % of all cases [40]. Agenesis of teeth appears to occur in women more frequently than in men [128, 132] and affects different tooth types with different frequencies.

The most common non-3rd molar permanent teeth affected are the mandibular 2nd premolars, maxillary lateral incisors, maxillary 2nd premolars, and mandibular incisors; however, the predominant tooth type missing may vary by ethnicity [6, 88, 132]. Additional phenotypes that may occur in the adult dentition with hypodontia include microdontia, peg-shaped tooth formation, displaced canines, rotated premolars and maxillary lateral incisors, tooth transpositions, taurodontism, infraocclusion, delayed tooth formation, delayed tooth eruption, and short root anomaly [6, 36, 128].

Nonsyndromic familial and sporadic dental agenesis is often transmitted as an AD trait with variable penetrance and variable expressivity, with the occurrence of peg-shaped lateral(s) instead of agenesis at times [6, 26, 154, 160, 167]. Certain forms of dental agenesis, however, exhibit autosomal recessive, X-linked, polygenic, or multifactorial models of inheritance [116]. Mutations in different genes involved in tooth development appear to result in dissimilar patterns in the number and type of teeth affected.

For example, *PAX9* mutations often show a nonsyndromic AD mode of inheritance for oligodontia with variable expressivity within families [46, 80, 89, 120, 155]. Molars in both dental arches are often affected by to *PAX9* mutations, while 2nd premolars in the maxilla arch appear to be affected more frequently than those located in the mandibular arch [19, 120]. In some cases, however, *PAX9* mutations can also affect mandibular central incisor and maxillary lateral incisor development, leading to peg-tooth formation or agenesis.

MSX1 gene mutations can lead to AD inheritance of 2nd-premolar and molar hypodontia or oligodontia [19, 31, 37, 86, 87, 93, 115, 127, 160, 169, 170]. In addition, mutations in the axis inhibitor 2 gene (*AXIN2*) have also been linked to oligodontia, often exhibited a similar pattern of affected teeth as *PAX9* mutations (i.e., molars, premolars, mandibular incisors > maxillary lateral incisors > canines) [19, 91]. The AXIN2 protein is a regulator of WNT and β-catenin signaling, so it is not surprising that mutations in the wingless-type MMTV integration site family, member 10A (*WNT10A*) gene have also been linked to hypodontia and oligodontia [1, 8, 113, 114, 150, 159].

Mutations with the ectodysplasin-A (*EDA*), EDA receptor (EDAR), and EDA receptor-associated death domain (*EDARADD*) genes have been shown to be involved in different forms of tooth agenesis [10, 19, 53, 121, 136, 143, 157, 158, 171]. Nonsyndromic EDA mutations appear to be X-linked traits exhibiting dominant or recessive modes of inheritance that largely affect incisor, canine, and premolar development [10, 53, 121, 136, 143, 157, 158, 171]. It is interesting to note that alteration in the *EDA* gene can also lead to a syndrome in humans termed X-linked hypohidrotic ectodermal dysplasia (XLHED), which presents with dental agenesis among other features. In studies of XLHED in dog and rodent models, replacement of the EDA recombinant protein has been shown to effectively correct key features (including dental development) of the disorder, when administered in the correct developmental window of time, offering hope that such therapies could be successful some day in humans [66]. A clinical trial is now under way to see if this is possible.

Duplication of the entire *RUNX2* gene in some individuals has been shown to lead to metopic craniosynostosis along with hypodontia/oligodontia (or tooth eruption problems), but hypodontia alone in others [50, 107, 111]. To date, mutations with at least seven different genes (*PAX9, EDA, MSX1, AXIN2, EDARADD, NEMO, and KRT17*) appear to be causal in nonsyndromic human oligodontia [141]. Other chromosomal locations and/or candidate genes thought to be involved in nonsyndromic hypodontia and/or oligodontia include transforming growth factor-alpha gene (*TNFA*) [28, 163], interferon regulatory factor 6 (*IRF6*) [164, 165], *FGF3* [162], fibroblast growth factor receptor 1 (*FGFR1*) [164], C2H2 zinc finger transcription factor 22 (*KROX-26/ZNF22*), and 10q11.2 [48, 97, 116]. An increased understanding of the various morphogenetic signaling pathways regulating tooth development should allow for induction of tooth development in areas of tooth agenesis [123].

5.5 Genetic Syndromes/Conditions That Are or May Be Associated with OTM Variation

Controlled human studies on OTM in various syndromes are essentially nonexistent. The most important limiting factor for tooth movement is the underlying condition of the bone [108]. Subjective observation, case reports, and animal studies give some insight into how various syndromes, conditions, and medications may affect OTM thought variation in connective tissue, bone physiology (mineralization, turnover, density), osteoclast differentiation/activation, and gingival fibromatosis (hyperplasia), which may be kept in mind by the orthodontist as they treat the patient in regard to mechanics including force level, expected length of treatment, and retention [9, 79, 148].

The dental history review for each patient should include a question on the loss of primary teeth early without trauma or other obvious reason. Not only may this indicate a medical problem, but could also foreshadow a concern about future OTM [57]. The following are a selected group of conditions or syndromes that could be involved:

Hypophosphatasia The disease is characterized by improper mineralization of bone caused by deficient (tissue nonspecific) alkaline phosphatase (*TNSALP/ALPL*) activity in the serum, liver, bone, and kidney.

The typical dental finding diagnostic of hypophosphatasia in children is premature exfoliation of the anterior primary teeth associated with deficient cementum. The loss of teeth in the young child may be spontaneous or may result from a slight trauma. Early exfoliation of the primary teeth is usually associated with the juvenile type of hypophosphatasia, although such a less severe history may be present in the adult type. Severe gingival inflammation will be absent, with loss of alveolar bone that may be limited to the anterior region. Treatment of patients with hypophosphatasia may be problematic because of the risk of permanent tooth loosening during OTM [102].

X-Linked Hypophosphatemic Rickets (X-Linked Hypophosphatemia) In addition to short stature and bowing of the lower extremities, there are often dental manifestations including apical radiolucencies, abscesses (that may result in premature exfoliation of teeth), and fistulas associated with pulp exposures in the primary and permanent teeth. The thin, hypomineralized enamel may abrade easily, exposing the pulp. Dental radiographs show rickety bone trabeculations and absent or abnormal lamina dura [57, 149].

There are other types of hypophosphatemia with overlapping clinical features and different modes of inheritance and genes involved. Generally, the more severe and earlier the onset, the more severe the dental manifestations will be. Vitamin D-deficient rickets however does not show the dental abnormalities found in X-linked hypophosphatemic rickets [57]. A relatively mild class II division 2 malocclusion case with severe anterior crowding and lack of mandibular growth was treated using a functional appliance, followed by the extraction of four premolars and the use of edgewise appliances, with no occurrence of root resorption or bone defect [82].

Early-Onset Periodontitis: Nonsyndromic and Syndromic, Including LAD Syndrome Types I and II Early-onset periodontitis may occur by itself (nonsyndromic) or as a part of a syndrome. For example, leukocyte adhesion deficiency (LAD) type I and type II are autosomal recessive disorders of the leukocyte adhesion cascade, with type I having an increased susceptibility for severe infections and early-onset (prepubertal) periodontitis [109]. The severity of the general infectious episodes is much milder LAD type II than those observed in LAD type I, although there is chronic severe periodontitis. Furthermore, patients with LAD type II present other abnormal features, such as growth and mental delay [43].

OTM into previously affected areas to correct crowding or anteroposterior discrepancies or reduce bimaxillary protrusion has been reported to be successful after a healing period following extractions secondary to periodontal disease. In addition, it has been claimed that after orthodontic space closure bony contours and attachment levels on repositioned second and third molars will be superior to those possible if the affected first molars were retained and treated. Periodontal evaluations should be scheduled as often as orthodontic appointments to monitor the condition during tooth movement [106].

Papillon-Lefèvre Syndrome One of the many different types of palmoplantar keratoderma (thickened skin over the palms and soles of the feet that may appear to be darkened or "dirty") differs from the others by the occurrence of severe early-onset periodontitis with premature loss of some or all of the primary and permanent dentition, as a characteristic sign. Lateral cephalometric analysis of eight patients with Papillon-Lefèvre syndrome revealed a tendency toward a class III skeletal relationship with maxillary retrognathia, decreased lower facial height, retroclined mandibular incisors, and upper lip retrusion [20]. It has been reported that following a successful combined mechanical and antibiotic therapy of periodontitis associated with the Papillon-Lefèvre syndrome, moderate orthodontic tooth movements may be possible within a complex interdisciplinary treatment regimen [101].

Hajdu-Cheney Syndrome Hajdu-Cheney syndrome (HCS) is a heritable, rare disorder of bone metabolism, associated with acroosteolysis, short stature, distinctive craniofacial and skull changes, periodontitis, and premature tooth loss. A 22-year-old female presented with the characteristic clinical features of HCS, including short stature, small face, prominent epicanthal folds, thin lips, small mouth, and short hands. Tests for bone mineral density were indicative of osteoporosis. Cephalometric analysis revealed hypoplasia of the midface and increased cranial base angle; the maxilla and the mandible were set posteriorly. The sella turcica was enlarged, elongated, and wide open with slender clinoids [15]. The mandible may be underdeveloped as well as the maxilla and midface. Le Fort III maxillary distraction osteogenesis and advancement genioplasty followed by orthodontia have been successfully performed for the midfacial retrusion and to eliminate severe snoring during sleep in a case [144].

Ehlers-Danlos Syndromes The Ehlers-Danlos syndromes (EDS) are a heterogeneous group of heritable connective tissue disorders characterized by articular hypermobility, skin extensibility, and tissue fragility. Other manifestations, including periodontal disease, can vary according to type of EDS. Classification revision has gone from at least ten types most of which were designated by Roman numerals to six main types (plus "other forms") based primarily on the etiology of each type.

The new designations are (a) classical type (formally Gravis (EDS type I) and Mitis (EDS type II)), (b) hypermobility type (formally hypermobile (EDS type III)), (c) vascular type (formally arterial-ecchymotic (EDS type IV)), (d) kyphoscoliosis type (ocular-scoliotic (EDS type VI)), (e) arthrochalasia type (arthrochalasis multiplex congenita (EDS types VIIA and VIIB)), and (f) dermatosparaxis type (human dermatosparaxis (EDS type VIIC). Other forms include what have been known as X-linked EDS (EDS type V), periodontitis type (EDS type VIII), fibronectin-deficient EDS (EDS type X), familial hypermobility syndrome (EDS type XI), progeroid EDS, and other unspecified forms [18].

Dental concerns in EDS have been included hypermobility of the TMJ with an increased incidence of subluxation, fragile oral mucosa, early-onset periodontitis, high cusps and deep fissures on the crowns of the teeth, high incidence of enamel and dental fractures, stunted roots or dilacerations, coronal pulp stones, aberrant dentinal tubules, pulpal vascular lesions and denticles, increased rate of tooth movement in response to orthodontic forces, and increased need for and duration of orthodontic retention [122].

The results of a survey about the orthodontic and temporomandibular disorder experiences of patients with EDS and a control sample of patients without EDS indicated that the majority of those with EDS types I, III, and VI experienced difficulty in their orthodontic treatment. Those with EDS type II found it tolerable, with a 25 % split between easy and difficult. This compared with the control group that unanimously reported orthodontic treatment as being either easy or tolerable. Frequent subluxation of the TMJ was found in all patients with EDS. This is a particular problem in EDS type II, IV, V, and VI patients [122].

Although not exclusively, major periodontal concerns in EDS are primarily in the "periodontal" (type VIII) and the "vascular" (type IV) variants. In addition to early-onset periodontitis, the periodontal-type patients have variable hyperextensibility of the skin, ecchymotic pretibial (purple discoloration of the shin) lesions of the skin, variable bruising besides the pretibial ecchymosis, minimal to moderate joint hypermobility of the digits, and "cigarette-paper" scars (in which the skin looks thin and crinkled) [62, 94, 153]. The outcome of orthodontic treatment in at least two cases of periodontal-type EDS is the basis for the recommendation that these patients may be considered to be a high-risk group for orthodontia not only in respect to alveolar bone loss but also for EARR.

For example, prior to starting the orthodontic treatment, one patient had since the age of 5 years atrophic, hyperpigmented scars on his shins, as well as bruising from mild trauma. He reportedly had suffered from gingival bleeding for many years. Four first premolars had been extracted at the beginning of the orthodontic treatment. Unfortunately the periodontal status had deteriorated after orthodontic treatment had been started with fixed appliances [25, 81]. Bright red, edematous gingival tissue with obvious recession was documented in another patient with the periodontitis type, along with early loss of his primary teeth and a history of severe periodontal disease [112].

Early periodontal disease may also be found in patients with vascular-type EDS. This type has some overlap clinically with the periodontal type, as evidenced by the finding of skin hyperextensibility, ecchymotic pretibial lesions, easy bruisibility, cigarette-paper scares, joint hypermobility of the digits, pes planus (flat feet), and of special importance arterial and intestinal ruptures, the last two features being major characteristics for diagnosis and prognosis [62].

Gingival Fibromatosis (Hyperplasia) Generalized gingival enlargement can be caused by a variety of etiological factors. It can be inherited as a nonsyndromic trait (hereditary gingival fibromatosis, HGF), associated with other diseases characterizing a syndrome, or most commonly induced as a side effect of medications such as phenytoin, cyclosporine, or nifedipine. Regardless of the etiology, the increase in thickness and firmness of the overlying gingiva may impede and/or alter the course of dental eruption and possibly affect OTM. Interestingly its occurrence is coincident usually, but not always, with the eruption of teeth, particularly of the permanent dentition [33, 60, 156].

Excision of the hyperplastic tissue is indicated for esthetic or functional reasons, including facilitation of tooth eruption, OTM, and good oral hygiene. It has been recommended that gingivectomy should only be carried out in the areas where the orthodontic treatment is about to be, or has been, initiated in order to reduce the chance of gingival hypertrophy recurrence. Although an increase in gingivitis and gingival hypertrophy is associated with fixed orthodontic appliances secondary to food retention and being more of a challenge in oral hygiene, it has been stated that it is not clear if the additional oral hygiene burden from fixed orthodontic appliances increases the severity of the hyperplasia or its postsurgical recurrence. Regardless, monthly periodontal checkups with scaling and polishing as indicated are recommended to counteract gingival inflammation as needed and to maximize healthy OTM [32, 83].

Down Syndrome Results from trisomy of all or a large part of chromosome 21, occurring in 1/660 births. Periodontal disease is common in the older patient, especially in the anterior mandibular region. Paradoxically they may have fewer dental caries, although baby bottle caries may be a concern. The tongue is often positioned partially outside the mouth (particularly when young), giving the impression that it is enlarged, although it is likely to be a posture secondary to hypotonia of the tongue and the facial musculature and the relatively small size of the oral cavity [11, 57, 63].

It has been stated that almost all individuals with Down syndrome have a significant malocclusion and typically a maxillary hypoplasia class III with anterior open bite, often with hypodontia, tooth size discrepancy, and occasionally impacted or transposed teeth. Considerations in the treatment of individuals with Down syndrome include a two-phase or multiphase plan to assist in early correction of maxillary transverse deficiency and class III malocclusion.

As with any individual with developmental delay, they must be able to cooperate and tolerate the discomfort associated with braces and orthodontic procedures to be treated effectively [63, 117]. This is a case by case evaluation. Working with them may be effective after some initial difficulty, but sometimes it is just not possible. Some procedures may be done in the operating room, but obviously this is not practical on any continuing basis for orthodontic treatment.

Treatment considerations include taking impressions using quickset materials with flavors that may reduce the tendency to gag frequently experienced with Down syndrome patients, bonding brackets instead of banding, using a self-etching primer with a glass ionomer cement that can be used in the oral environment when it is difficult to maintain a dry field for several minutes at a time, using nickel-titanium wires when and for as long as possible allowing a longer interval between appointments, and using implants in treatment planning to replace agenic teeth and temporary anchorage devices to minimize the need for compliance [117].

Osteogenesis Imperfecta Osteogenesis imperfecta (OI) is a heterogeneous group of conditions affecting bone mass and fragility. It is a highly variable disease that is usually secondary to an abnormality in type I collagen synthesis or extracellular secretion. However, some OI patients with normal type I collagen apparently have mutations affecting other bone proteins. The hallmark sign of OI ("brittle bone disease") is an increased incidence or history of bone fracture, usually resulting from minimal if any trauma. There are associated craniofacial and dental manifestations that may include dentinogenesis imperfecta, a hypoplastic maxilla, and hypodontia, among others. Variable expression of dentin developmental defects has been documented, with approximately one-fourth to three-fourths of the cases showing some manifestation of dentinogenesis imperfecta, depending to some degree on the type of OI [61].

There are several types of OI, based on phenotype (clinical picture) and to some degree genotype. Taking all the different types and manifestations of OI as a group, the incidence is probably between 1 in 5000–10,000 individuals [27]. Documentation of histological dentin abnormalities, in clinically and radiographically normal teeth, indicates that the effect on dentin development is a continuum. In addition to dentinogenesis imperfecta, the presence of additional dental and craniofacial manifestations has been documented: attrition of teeth and tooth fracture (associated with dentinogenesis imperfecta), thistle-shaped pulp chambers, apically extended pulp chambers (resembling taurodontism), denticles, maxillary lateral incisor invagination, gemination, odontoma, periapical radiolucencies in noncarious teeth, class III malocclusion (more common than class II malocclusion), maxillary hypoplasia, anterior and posterior crossbite, anterior and posterior open bite that tends to worsen with age, hypodontia, supernumerary teeth (rare), variation in dental development, mandibular cysts (rare), and lack of eruption (or ectopic eruption) of the first and/or second permanent molars [98–100, 103, 124, 130, 145].

Bone continues to form during the growth period in patients with OI [78]. Although all patients with OI are said to be osteoporotic, it has not been determined if bone mineralization patterns in the lumbar spine or other locations correlate well with those of the craniofacies, so bone mineral density determinations in other parts of the body may not be informative for orthognathic surgery and other treatment such as OTM [124]. In general rapid palatal expansion and tooth movement are not a problem, although the teeth may seem relatively loose after debonding, so immediate and long-term retention is advised. Care should be taken when debonding brackets from teeth with dentinogenesis imperfecta to minimize the chance of their fracture and chipping. Although banding of teeth may be contemplated if some teeth are already chipped or fractures prior to initiating orthodontic treatment, prudence may indicate no orthodontic attachments on those teeth and possibly some restorative coverage.

The variability of the facial bone quality is so great that prediction of orthognathic surgery outcome can be uncertain until the surgeon actually makes the osteotomies and places the surgical fasteners. In addition, patients with OI have additional general anesthesia and possible bleeding concerns of which the anesthesiologist and surgeon should be aware.

In summary by the "classic" OI types:

OI type I: Patients can receive orthodontic treatment as their treatment response to orthodontic forces is fairly similar to a non-affected population [61], and their treatment is manageable in private orthodontic offices [30].

Types III and IV: These patients typically present with more complicated challenges. They are often in a wheelchair, with more severe craniofacial deformities, especially the class III lateral open-bite malocclusions found in a great proportion of these patients. Orthodontic tooth movement should be expected to be markedly slowed due to the lack of bone resorption *if* bisphosphonates are being, or have recently been, used in these patients, as it is common for them to be on i.v. infusion in children and injections or oral intake in adults [61]. Clinically, the effect on the rate of OTM is variable and may be particularly resistant to extrusion to treat posterior open bites in the posterior dentition of OI type IV or III patients [138].

Cleidocranial Dysplasia (Dysostosis) This AD condition is characterized by variable agenesis or hypoplasia of the clavicles (allowing the shoulders to be rolled to the body midline in the more severe cases), delayed and imperfect ossification of the cranium (with variable persistence of open fontanels and sutures), moderately short stature, and a variety of other skeletal abnormalities, although variable expressivity may be seen even in affected members of the same family [44, 49].

The maxillary hypoplasia may result in a relative mandibular protrusion. The dental manifestations are a delayed exfoliation of primary teeth, a lack of or delayed eruption of the permanent dentition that may appear without radiography to be hypodontia, and multiple supernumerary teeth [44]. Patients with cleidocranial dysostosis (CCD) benefit from a team approach with good cooperation and communication within the team and with the patient and family [44]. As with any patient with a hypoplastic/retrusive maxilla, timing of a dentofacial orthopedic intervention to bring the maxilla ventrally is critical, usually before the age of 10 years of age depending on skeletal maturation [32, 102]. Further orthodontic treatment and surgery may be required following the pubertal growth spurt. Although there are an abundance of teeth present, sometimes they cannot be moved or placed in an acceptable position, which may necessitate prosthetics with or without surgery as needed.

Although several methods, surgical and/or prosthetic, have been put forth for the treatment of CCD, the "Jerusalem" protocol has been recommended as an initial consideration. This involves two surgeries (anterior and posterior) under general anesthesia at the stage when the root development of unerupted teeth is at least two-thirds of their final estimated length. The first surgery is performed at the chronological age of 10–12 years, with which the usual dental development delay in CCD corresponds to a dental age of 7–8 years. In addition to the extraction of deciduous incisors and supernumerary unerupted teeth in both arches, unerupted permanent incisors are exposed and have attachments bonded to them, followed by primary closure of the surgical flaps. The immature posterior permanent teeth are not exposed or their dental follicles disturbed at this stage.

In the second operation (chronological age of at least 13 years; dental age of 10–11 years), deciduous canines and molars are extracted, permanent canines and premolars are exposed in both arches, attachments are bonded, and the surgical flap is closed. Care should be taken in the extraction of supernumerary unerupted teeth and the exposure of permanent unerupted teeth in order to maintain the integrity of vestibular and lingual/palatal bone plates. Bone is only removed around the crowns of the permanent teeth as needed for the bonding of attachments. In order to encourage healing by primary intention, the flap is repositioned so as to completely cover the wound, without compresses/pressure. Traction is placed by the application of low extrusion forces using rigid upper and lower arches and anterior box elastic between the two arches to oppose the possible distortions caused by the excess of space in the arch and the resistance to extrusion. Further details of the treatment protocol may be found in the cited papers by Becker et al. [16, 17, 34].

5.6 In Summary

Various types of genetic factors can have a significant effect on OTM, EARR, primary failure of eruption (PFE), and dental agenesis. The clinician should be aware of these factors, particularly the possible inverse relationship between velocity of OTM and EARR, the resulting ankylosis when attempting to extrude teeth affected by PFE, the variety and other dental developmental anomalies associated with dental agenesis, and the effect of some syndromes on OTM and other aspects of orthodontic treatment. Until further advances are made in genetic testing and understanding, the results in relation to orthodontic treatment, the careful examination of the patient, awareness of the patient's developmental and family history, and monitoring of the progress of treatment are the clinician's best instruments to deal with these genetic factors in the treatment of their patients.

References

1. Abdalla EM, Mostowska A, Jagodziński PP, Dwidar K, Ismail SR. A novel *WNT10A* mutation causes non-syndromic hypodontia in an Egyptian family. Arch Oral Biol. 2014;59:722–8.
2. Afify AR, Zawawi KH. The prevalence of dental anomalies in the Western region of saudi arabia. ISRN Dent. 2012;2012:837270.
3. Al-Qawasmi RA, Hartsfield Jr JK, Everett ET, Flury L, Liu L, Foroud TM, Macri JV, Roberts WE. Genetic predisposition to external apical root resorption. Am J Orthod Dentofacial Orthop. 2003;123:242–52.
4. Al-Qawasmi RA, Hartsfield Jr JK, Everett ET, Flury L, Liu L, Foroud TM, Macri JV, Roberts WE. Genetic predisposition to external apical root resorption in orthodontic patients: linkage of chromosome-18 marker. J Dent Res. 2003;82:356–60.
5. Al-Qawasmi RA, Hartsfield Jr JK, Everett ET, Weaver MR, Foroud TM, Roberts WE. Root resorption associated with orthodontic force in IL-1Beta knockout mouse. J Musculoskelet Neuronal Interact. 2004;4:383–5.
6. Arte S, Nieminen P, Apajalahti S, Haavikko K, Thesleff I, Pirinen S. Characteristics of incisor-premolar hypodontia in families. J Dent Res. 2001;80:1445–50.
7. Arte S, Pirinen S. Hypodontia [Online]. 2004. Available: http://www.orpha.net/data/patho/GB/uk-hypodontia.pdf.
8. Arzoo PS, Klar J, Bergendal B, Norderyd J, Dahl N. *WNT10A* mutations account for (1/4) of population-based isolated oligodontia and show phenotypic correlations. Am J Med Genet A. 2014;164A:353–9.
9. Ashcraft MB, Southard KA, Tolley EA. The effect of corticosteroid-induced osteoporosis on orthodontic tooth movement. Am J Orthod Dentofacial Orthop. 1992;102:310–9.
10. Ayub M, Ur-Rehman F, Yasinzai M, Ahmad W. A novel missense mutation in the ectodysplasin-A (*EDA*) gene underlies X-linked recessive nonsyndromic hypodontia. Int J Dermatol. 2010;49:1399–402.
11. Babic M, Scepan I, micic M. Comparative cephalometric analysis in patients with X-chromosome aneuploidy. Arch Oral Biol. 1993;38:179–83.
12. Baltimore D. Our genome unveiled. Nature. 2001;409:814–6.
13. Bastos Lages EM, Drummond AF, Pretti H, Costa FO, Lages EJ, Gontijo AI, Miranda Cota LO, Brito Jr RB. Association of functional gene polymorphism IL-1beta in patients with external apical root resorption. Am J Orthod Dentofacial Orthop. 2009;136:542–6.
14. Baumrind S, Korn EL, Boyd RL. Apical root resorption in orthodontically treated adults. Am J Orthod Dentofacial Orthop. 1996;110:311–20.
15. Bazopoulou-Kyrkanidou E, Vrahopoulos TP, Eliades G, Vastardis H, Tosios K, Vrotsos IA. Periodontitis associated with Hajdu-Cheney syndrome. J Periodontol. 2007;78:1831–8.
16. Becker A, Lustmann J, Shteyer A. Cleidocranial dysplasia: part 1 – general principles of the orthodontic and surgical treatment modality. Am J Orthod Dentofacial Orthop. 1997;111:28–33.
17. Becker A, Shteyer A, Bimstein E, Lustmann J. Cleidocranial dysplasia: part 2 – treatment protocol for the orthodontic and surgical modality. Am J Orthod Dentofacial Orthop. 1997;111:173–83.
18. Beighton P, De Paepe A, Steinmann B, Tsipouras P, Wenstrup RJ. Ehlers-Danlos syndromes: revised nosology, Villefranche, 1997. Ehlers-Danlos National Foundation (USA) and Ehlers-Danlos Support Group (UK). Am J Med Genet. 1998;77:31–7.
19. Bergendal B, Klar J, Stecksen-Blicks C, Norderyd J, Dahl N. Isolated oligodontia associated with mutations in EDARADD, AXIN2, MSX1, and PAX9 genes. Am J Med Genet A. 2011;155A:1616–22.
20. Bindayel NA, Ullbro C, Suri L, Al-Farra E. Cephalometric findings in patients with Papillon-Lefevre syndrome. Am J Orthod Dentofacial Orthop. 2008;134:138–44.

21. Brezniak N, Wasserstein A. Root resorption after orthodontic treatment: part 1. Literature review. Am J Orthod Dentofacial Orthop. 1993;103:62–6.
22. Brezniak N, Wasserstein A. Root resorption after orthodontic treatment: part 2. Literature review. Am J Orthod Dentofacial Orthop. 1993;103:138–46.
23. Brook AH. Multilevel complex interactions between genetic, epigenetic and environmental factors in the aetiology of anomalies of dental development. Arch Oral Biol. 2009;54 Suppl 1:S3–17.
24. Brook AH, Elcock C, Al-Sharood MH, Mckeown HF, Khalaf K, Smith RN. Further studies of a model for the etiology of anomalies of tooth number and size in humans. Connect Tissue Res. 2002;43:289–95.
25. Buckel T, Zaenglein AL. what syndrome is this? ehlers-danlos syndrome type viii. Pediatr Dermatol. 2007;24:189–91.
26. Burzynski NJ, Escobar VH. Classification and genetics of numeric anomalies of dentition. Birth Defects Orig Artic Ser. 1983;19:95–106.
27. Byers PH, Steiner RD. Osteogenesis imperfecta. Annu Rev Med. 1992;43:269–82.
28. Callahan N, Modesto A, Deeley K, Meira R, Vieira AR. Transforming growth factor-alfa gene (*TGFA*), human tooth agenesis, and evidence of segmental uniparental isodisomy. Eur J Oral Sci. 2009;117:20–6.
29. Carter K, Worthington S. Morphologic and demographic predictors of third molar agenesis: a systematic review and meta-analysis. J Dent Res. 2015;94:886–94.
30. Cassidy SB, Allanson JE. Management of genetic syndromes. New York: Wiley; 2010.
31. Chishti MS, Muhammad D, Haider M, Ahmad W. A novel missense mutation in MSX1 underlies autosomal recessive oligodontia with associated dental anomalies in Pakistani families. J Hum Genet. 2006;51:872–8.
32. Clocheret K, Dekeyser C, Carels C, Willems G. Idiopathic gingival hyperplasia and orthodontic treatment: a case report. J Orthod. 2003;30:13–9.
33. Coletta RD, Graner E. Hereditary gingival fibromatosis: a systematic review. J Periodontol. 2006;77:753–64.
34. D'alessandro G, Tagariello T, Piana G. Craniofacial changes and treatment of the stomatognathic system in subjects with Cleidocranial dysplasia. Eur J Paediatr Dent. 2010;11: 39–43.
35. Danis V, Millington M, Hyland V, Grennan D. Cytokine production by normal human monocytes: inter-subject variation and relationship to an IL-1 receptor antagonist (IL-1Ra) gene polymorphism. Clin Exp Immunol. 1995;99:303.
36. DE Coster PJ, Marks LA, Martens LC, Huysseune A. Dental agenesis: genetic and clinical perspectives. J Oral Pathol Med. 2009;38:1–17.
37. DE Muynck S, Schollen E, Matthijs G, Verdonck A, Devriendt K, Carels C. A novel MSX1 mutation in hypodontia. Am J Med Genet A. 2004;128A:401–3.
38. Decker E, Stellzig-Eisenhauer A, Fiebig BS, Rau C, Kress W, Saar K, Ruschendorf F, Hubner N, Grimm T, Weber BH. PTHR1 loss-of-function mutations in familial, nonsyndromic primary failure of tooth eruption. Am J Hum Genet. 2008;83:781–6.
39. Deshields RW. A study of root resorption in treated Class II, Division I malocclusions. Angle Orthod. 1969;39:231–45.
40. Dhanrajani PJ. Hypodontia: Etiology, clinical features, and management. Quintessence Int. 2002;33:294–302.
41. Dinarello CA. Biologic basis for interleukin-1 in disease. Blood. 1996;87:2095–147.
42. Enlow DH. Growth of the Craniofacial Skeleton. In: Riolo ML, Cangialosi TJ, Hartsfield Jr JK, Lipp MJ, editors. Essentials for orthodontic practice. 3rd ed. Ann Arbor: Essential Press; 2012.
43. Etzioni A, Tonetti M. Leukocyte adhesion deficiency II-from A to almost Z. Immunol Rev. 2000;178:138–47.
44. Farronato G, Maspero C, Farronato D, Gioventu S. Orthodontic treatment in a patient with cleidocranial dysostosis. Angle Orthod. 2009;79:178–85.

45. Fontana ML, de Souza CM, Bernardino JF, Hoette F, Hoette ML, Thum L, Ozawa TO, Capelozza Filho L, Olandoski M, Trevilatto PC. Association analysis of clinical aspects and vitamin D receptor gene polymorphism with external apical root resorption in orthodontic patients. Am J Orthod Dentofacial Orthop. 2012;142:339–47.
46. Frazier-Bowers SA, Guo DC, Cavender A, Xue L, Evans B, King T, Milewicz D, D'souza RN. A novel mutation in human PAX9 causes molar oligodontia. J Dent Res. 2002;81: 129–33.
47. Frazier-Bowers SA, Simmons D, Wright JT, Proffit WR, Ackerman JL. Primary failure of eruption and PTH1R: the importance of a genetic diagnosis for orthodontic treatment planning. Am J Orthod Dentofacial Orthop. 2010;137(160):e1–7; discussion 160–1.
48. Gao Y, Kobayashi H, Ganss B. The human KROX-26/ZNF22 gene is expressed at sites of tooth formation and maps to the locus for permanent tooth agenesis (He-Zhao deficiency). J Dent Res. 2003;82:1002–7.
49. Golan I, Baumert U, Wagener H, Preising M, Lorenz B, Niederdellmann H, Mussig D. Evidence of intrafamilial variability of CBFA1/RUNX2 expression in cleidocranial dysplasia – a family study. J Orofac Orthop. 2002;63:190–8.
50. Greives MR, Odessey EA, Waggoner DJ, Shenaq DS, Aradhya S, Mitchell A, Whitcomb E, Warshawsky N, He TC, Reid RR. RUNX2 quadruplication: additional evidence toward a new form of syndromic craniosynostosis. J Craniofac Surg. 2013;24:126–9.
51. Gülden N, Eggermann T, Zerres K, Beer M, Meinelt A, Diedrich P. Interleukin-1 polymorphisms in relation to external apical root resorption (EARR). J Orofac Orthop. 2009;70: 20–38.
52. Haga S, Nakaoka H, Yamaguchi T, Yamamoto K, Kim YI, Samoto H, Ohno T, Katayama K, Ishida H, Park SB, Kimura R, Maki K, Inoue I. A genome-wide association study of third molar agenesis in Japanese and Korean populations. J Hum Genet. 2013;58:799–803.
53. Han D, Gong Y, Wu H, Zhang X, Yan M, Wang X, Qu H, Feng H, Song S. Novel EDA mutation resulting in X-linked non-syndromic hypodontia and the pattern of EDA-associated isolated tooth agenesis. Eur J Med Genet. 2008;51:536–46.
54. Harris EF, Butler ML. Patterns of incisor root resorption before and after orthodontic correction in cases with anterior open bites. Am J Orthod Dentofacial Orthop. 1992;101:112–9.
55. Harris EF, Kineret SE, Tolley EA. A heritable component for external apical root resorption in patients treated orthodontically. Am J Orthod Dentofacial Orthop. 1997;111:301–9.
56. Harris EF, Robinson QC, Woods MA. An analysis of causes of apical root resorption in patients not treated orthodontically. Quintessence Int. 1993;24:417–28.
57. Hartsfield Jr JK. Premature exfoliation of teeth in childhood and adolescence. Adv Pediatr. 1994;41:453–70.
58. Hartsfield Jr JK. Pathways in external apical root resorption associated with orthodontia. Orthod Craniofac Res. 2009;12:236–42.
59. Hartsfield Jr JK. Personalized orthodontics, limitations and possibilities in practice. In: Krishnan V, Davidovitch Z, editors. Biological mechanisms of tooth movement. 2nd ed. Chichester/West Sussex/Ames/Iowa: Wiley; 2015.
60. Hartsfield Jr JK, Bixler D, Hazen RH. Gingival fibromatosis with sensorineural hearing loss: an autosomal dominant trai. Am J Med Genet. 1985;22:623–7.
61. Hartsfield Jr JK, Hohlt WF, Roberts WE. Orthodontic treatment and orthognathic surgery for patients with osteogenesis imperfecta. Semin Orthod. 2006;12:254–71.
62. Hartsfield Jr JK, Kousseff BG. Phenotypic overlap of Ehlers-Danlos syndrome types IV and VIII. Am J Med Genet. 1990;37:465–70.
63. Hennequin M, Faulks D, Veyrune JL, Bourdiol P. Significance of oral health in persons with down syndrome: a literature review. Dev Med Child Neurol. 1999;41:275–83.
64. Horiuchi A, Hotokezaka H, Kobayashi K. Correlation between cortical plate proximity and apical root resorption. Am J Orthod Dentofacial Orthop. 1998;114:311–8.
65. Hurme M, Santtila S. IL-1 receptor antagonist (IL-1Ra) plasma levels are co-ordinately regulated by both IL-1Ra and IL-1β genes. Eur J Immunol. 1998;28:2598–602.

66. Huttner K. Future developments in XLHED treatment approaches. Am J Med Genet A. 2014;164A:2433–6.
67. Iglesias-Linares A. Postorthodontic external root resorption is associated with IL1 receptor antagonist gene variations. Oral Dis. 2011;18:198–205.
68. Iglesias-Linares A, Yanez-Vico RM, Ballesta S, Ortiz-Ariza E, Mendoza-Mendoza A, Perea E, Solano-Reina E. Interleukin 1 gene cluster SNPs (rs1800587, rs1143634) influences post-orthodontic root resorption in endodontic and their contralateral vital control teeth differently. Int Endod J. 2012;45:1018–26.
69. Iglesias-Linares A, Yanez-Vico RM, Ballesta-Mudarra S, Ortiz-Ariza E, Mendoza-Mendoza A, Perea-Perez E, Moreno-Fernandez AM, Solano-Reina E. Interleukin 1 receptor antagonist (IL1RN) genetic variations condition post-orthodontic external root resorption in endodontically-treated teeth. Histol Histopathol. 2013;28:767–73.
70. Iglesias-Linares A, Yanez-Vico R, Ballesta-Mudarra S, Ortiz-Ariza E, Ortega-Rivera H, Mendoza-Mendoza A, Solano-Reina E, Perea-Perez E. Postorthodontic external root resorption is associated with IL1 receptor antagonist gene variations. Oral Dis. 2012;18:198–205.
71. Iglesias-Linares A, Yanez-Vico RM, Moreno-Fernandez AM, Mendoza-Mendoza A, Orce-Romero A, Solano-Reina E. Osteopontin gene SNPs (rs9138, rs11730582) mediate susceptibility to external root resorption in orthodontic patients. Oral Dis. 2014;20:307–12.
72. Iglesias-Linares A, Yanez-Vico RM, Ortiz-Ariza E, Ballesta S, Mendoza-Mendoza A, Perea E, Solano-Reina E. Postorthodontic external root resorption in root-filled teeth is influenced by interleukin-1beta polymorphism. J Endod. 2012;38:283–7.
73. Iwasaki L, Crouch L, Reinhardt R, Nickel J. The velocity of human orthodontic tooth movement is related to stress magnitude, growth status, and the ratio of cytokines in gingival crevicular fluid. Biological mechanisms of tooth movement and craniofacial adaptation. Boston: Harvard Society for the Advancement of Orthodontics; 2004. p. 137–47.
74. Iwasaki LR, Crouch LD, Tutor A, Gibson S, Hukmani N, Marx DB, Nickel JC. Tooth movement and cytokines in gingival crevicular fluid and whole blood in growing and adult subjects. Am J Orthod Dentofacial Orthop. 2005;128:483–91.
75. Iwasaki L, Crouch L, Nickel J. Genetic factors and tooth movement. Semin Orthod. 2008;14:135–45. Elsevier.
76. Iwasaki LR, Gibson CS, Crouch LD, Marx DB, Pandey JP, Nickel JC. Speed of tooth movement is related to stress and IL-1 gene polymorphisms. Am J Orthod Dentofacial Orthop. 2006;130:698.e1–9.
77. Iwasaki LR, Haack JE, Nickel JC, Morton J. Human tooth movement in response to continuous stress of low magnitude. Am J Orthod Dentofacial Orthop. 2000;117:175–83.
78. Jones SJ, Glorieux FH, Travers R, Boyde A. The microscopic structure of bone in normal children and patients with osteogenesis imperfecta: a survey using backscattered electron imaging. Calcif Tissue Int. 1999;64:8–17.
79. Kalia S, Melsen B, Verna C. Tissue reaction to orthodontic tooth movement in acute and chronic corticosteroid treatment*. Orthod Craniofac Res. 2004;7:26–34.
80. Kapadia H, Frazier-Bowers S, Ogawa T, D'souza RN. Molecular characterization of a novel PAX9 missense mutation causing posterior tooth agenesis. Eur J Hum Genet. 2006;14: 403–9.
81. Karrer S, Landthaler M, Schmalz G. Ehlers-Danlos syndrome type VIII with severe periodontitis and apical root resorption after orthodontic treatment. Acta Derm Venereol. 2000; 80:56–7.
82. Kawakami M, Takano-Yamamoto T. Orthodontic treatment of a patient with hypophosphatemic vitamin D-resistant rickets. ASDC J Dent Child. 1997;64:395–9.
83. Kelekis-Cholakis A, Wiltshire WA, Birek C. Treatment and long-term follow-up of a patient with hereditary gingival fibromatosis: a case report. J Can Dent Assoc. 2002;68:290–4.
84. Kerekes-Máthé B, Brook AH, Mártha K, Székely M, Smith RN. Mild Hypodontia is associated with smaller tooth dimensions and cusp numbers than in controls. Arch Oral Biol. 2015;60:1442–9.

85. Khalaf K, Miskelly J, Voge E, Macfarlane TV. Prevalence of hypodontia and associated factors: a systematic review and meta-analysis. J Orthod. 2014;41:299–316.
86. Kim JW, Simmer JP, Lin BP, Hu JC. Novel MSX1 frameshift causes autosomal-dominant oligodontia. J Dent Res. 2006;85:267–71.
87. Kimura M, Machida J, Yamaguchi S, Shibata A, Tatematsu T, Miyachi H, Jezewski PA, Nakayama A, Higashi Y, Shimozato K, Tokita Y. Novel nonsense mutation in MSX1 in familial nonsyndromic oligodontia: subcellular localization and role of homeodomain/MH4. Eur J Oral Sci. 2014;122:15–20.
88. Kirzioglu Z, Koseler Sentut T, Ozay Erturk MS, Karayilmaz H. Clinical features of hypodontia and associated dental anomalies: a retrospective study. Oral Dis. 2005;11: 399–404.
89. Klein ML, Nieminen P, Lammi L, Niebuhr E, Kreiborg S. Novel mutation of the initiation codon of PAX9 causes oligodontia. J Dent Res. 2005;84:43–7.
90. Kurol J, Owman-Moll P, Lundgren D. Time-related root resorption after application of a controlled continuous orthodontic force. Am J Orthod Dentofacial Orthop. 1996;110: 303–10.
91. Lammi L, Arte S, Somer M, Jarvinen H, Lahermo P, Thesleff I, Pirinen S, Nieminen P. Mutations in AXIN2 cause familial tooth agenesis and predispose to colorectal cancer. Am J Hum Genet. 2004;74:1043–50.
92. Lerner UH, Modéer T, Krekmanova L, Claesson R, Rasmussen L. Gingival crevicular fluid from patients with periodontitis contains bone resorbing activity. Eur J Oral Sci. 1998; 106:778–87.
93. Lidral AC, Reising BC. The role of MSX1 in human tooth agenesis. J Dent Res. 2002; 81:274–8.
94. Linch DC, Acton CH. Ehlers-Danlos syndrome presenting with juvenile destructive periodontitis. Br Dent J. 1979;147:95–6.
95. Linge L, Linge BO. Patient characteristics and treatment variables associated with apical root resorption during orthodontic treatment. Am J Orthod Dentofacial Orthop. 1991;99: 35–43.
96. Linhartova P, Cernochova P, Izakovicova Holla L. IL1 gene polymorphisms in relation to external apical root resorption concurrent with orthodontia. Oral Dis. 2013;19:262–70.
97. Liu W, Wang H, Zhao S, Zhao W, Bai S, Zhao Y, Xu S, Wu C, Huang W, Chen Z, Feng G, He L. The novel gene locus for agenesis of permanent teeth (He-Zhao deficiency) maps to chromosome 10q11.2. J Dent Res. 2001;80:1716–20.
98. Lukinmaa PL, Ranta H, Ranta K, Kaitila I, Hietanen J. Dental findings in osteogenesis imperfecta: II Dysplastic and other developmental defects. J Craniofac Genet Dev Biol. 1987;7: 127–35.
99. Lukinmaa PL, Ranta H, Ranta K, Kaitila I. Dental findings in osteogenesis imperfecta: I Occurrence and expression of type I dentinogenesis imperfecta. J Craniofac Genet Dev Biol. 1987;7:115–25.
100. Lund AM, Jensen BL, Nielsen LA, Skovby F. Dental manifestations of osteogenesis imperfecta and abnormalities of collagen I metabolism. J Craniofac Genet Dev Biol. 1998;18: 30–7.
101. Lux CJ, Kugel B, Komposch G, Pohl S, Eickholz P. Orthodontic treatment in a patient with Papillon-Lefevre syndrome. J Periodontol. 2005;76:642–50.
102. Macfarlane JD, Swart JG. Dental aspects of hypophosphatasia: a case report, family study, and literature review. Oral Surg Oral Med Oral Pathol. 1989;67:521–6.
103. Malmgren B, Norgren S. Dental aberrations in children and adolescents with osteogenesis imperfecta. Acta Odontol Scand. 2002;60:65–71.
104. Massler M, Malone AJ. Root resorption in human permanent teeth: a Roentgenographic study. Am J Orthod. 1954;40:19–33.
105. Massler M, Perreault JG. Root resorption in the permanent teeth of young adults. J Dent Child. 1954;21:158–64.

106. Mclain JB, Proffit WR, Davenport RH. Adjunctive orthodontic therapy in the treatment of juvenile periodontitis: report of a case and review of the literature. Am J Orthod. 1983;83: 290–8.
107. Mefford HC, Shafer N, Antonacci F, Tsai JM, Park SS, Hing AV, Rieder MJ, Smyth MD, Speltz ML, Eichler EE, Cunningham ML. Copy number variation analysis in single-suture craniosynostosis: multiple rare variants including RUNX2 duplication in two cousins with metopic craniosynostosis. Am J Med Genet A. 2010;152A:2203–10.
108. Melsen B. What are the limits of orthodontic treatment? Adult Orthodon. 2012;382–3.
109. Meyle J, Gonzales JR. Influences of systemic diseases on periodontitis in children and adolescents. Periodontol 2000. 2001;26:92–112.
110. Mina M, Kollar EJ. The induction of odontogenesis in non-dental mesenchyme combined with early murine mandibular arch epithelium. Arch Oral Biol. 1987;32:123–7.
111. Molin A, Lopez-Cazaux S, Pichon O, Vincent M, Isidor B, LE Caignec C. Patients with isolated oligo/hypodontia caused by RUNX2 duplication. Am J Med Genet A. 2015;167: 1386–90.
112. Moore MM, Votava JM, Orlow SJ, Schaffer JV. Ehlers-Danlos syndrome type VIII: Periodontitis, easy bruising, marfanoid habitus, and distinctive facies. J Am Acad Dermatol. 2006;55:S41–5.
113. Mostowska A, Biedziak B, Zadurska M, Dunin-Wilczynska I, Lianeri M, Jagodzinski PP. Nucleotide variants of genes encoding components of the Wnt signalling pathway and the risk of non-syndromic tooth agenesis. Clin Genet. 2013;84:429–40.
114. Mostowska A, Biedziak B, Zadurska M, Matuszewska-Trojan S, Jagodzinski PP. *WNT10A* coding variants and maxillary lateral incisor agenesis with associated dental anomalies. Eur J Oral Sci. 2015;123:1–8.
115. Mostowska A, Biedziak B, Trzeciak WH. A novel c.581C>T transition localized in a highly conserved homeobox sequence of MSX1: is it responsible for oligodontia? J Appl Genet. 2006;47:159–64.
116. Mostowska A, Kobielak A, Biedziak B, Trzeciak WH. Novel mutation in the paired box sequence of PAX9 gene in a sporadic form of oligodontia. Eur J Oral Sci. 2003;111: 272–6.
117. Musich DR. Orthodontic intervention and patients with down syndrome. Angle Orthod. 2006;76:734–5.
118. Nayak BN, Galil KA, Wiltshire W, Lekic PC. Molecular biology of orthodontic tooth movement. J Dent Oral Health. 2013;1:1–6.
119. Newman WG. Possible etiologic factors in external root resorption. Am J Orthod. 1975;67: 522–39.
120. Nieminen P, Arte S, Tanner D, Paulin L, Alaluusua S, Thesleff I, Pirinen S. Identification of a nonsense mutation in the PAX9 gene in molar oligodontia. Eur J Hum Genet. 2001;9: 743–6.
121. Nikopensius T, Annilo T, Jagomägi T, Gilissen C, Kals M, Krjutškov K, Mägi R, Eelmets M, Gerst-Talas U, Remm M, Saag M, Hoischen A, Metspalu A. Non-syndromic tooth agenesis associated with a nonsense mutation in ectodysplasin-a (EDA). J Dent Res. 2013;92: 507–11.
122. Norton LA, Assael LA. Orthodontic and temporomandibular joint considerations in treatment of patients with Ehlers-Danlos syndrome. Am J Orthod Dentofacial Orthop. 1997;111: 75–84.
123. Nuckolls GH, Shum L, Slavkin HC. Progress toward understanding craniofacial malformations. Cleft Palate Craniofac J. 1999;36:12–26.
124. O'connell AC, Marini JC. Evaluation of oral problems in an osteogenesis imperfecta population. Oral Surg Oral Med Oral Pathol Oral Radiol Endod. 1999;87:189–96.
125. Owman-Moll P, Kurol J, Lundgren D. Continuous versus interrupted continuous orthodontic force related to early tooth movement and root resorption. Angle Orthod. 1995;65:395–401; discussion 401–2.

126. Parker RJ, Harris EF. Directions of orthodontic tooth movements associated with external apical root resorption of the maxillary central incisor. Am J Orthod Dentofacial Orthop. 1998;114:677–83.
127. Pawlowska E, Janik-Papis K, Wisniewska-Jarosinska M, Szczepanska J, Blasiak J. Mutations in the human homeobox MSX1 gene in the congenital lack of permanent teeth. Tohoku J Exp Med. 2009;217:307–12.
128. Peck L, Peck S, Attia Y. Maxillary canine-first premolar transposition, associated dental anomalies and genetic basis. Angle Orthod. 1993;63:99–109; discussion 110.
129. Pereira S, Lavado N, Nogueira L, Lopez M, Abreu J, Silva H. Polymorphisms of genes encoding P2X7R, IL-1B, OPG and RANK in orthodontic-induced apical root resorption. Oral Dis. 2014;20:659–67.
130. Petersen K, Wetzel WE. Recent findings in classification of osteogenesis imperfecta by means of existing dental symptoms. ASDC J Dent Child. 1998;65(305–9):354.
131. Pociot F, Mølvig J, Wogensen L, Worsaae H, Nerup J. A Taql polymorphism in the human interleukin-1β (IL-1β) gene correlates with IL-1β secretion in vitro. Eur J Clin Invest. 1992;22:396–402.
132. Polder BJ, Van't Hof MA, Van Der Linden FP, Kuijpers-Jagtman AM. A meta-analysis of the prevalence of dental agenesis of permanent teeth. Community Dent Oral Epidemiol. 2004;32: 217–26.
133. Proffit WR, Frazier-Bowers SA. Mechanism and control of tooth eruption: overview and clinical implications. Orthod Craniofac Res. 2009;12:59–66.
134. Proffit WR, Vig KW. Primary failure of eruption: a possible cause of posterior open-bite. Am J Orthod. 1981;80:173–90.
135. Raghoebar GM, Boering G, Jansen HW, Vissink A. Secondary retention of permanent molars: a histologic study. J Oral Pathol Med. 1989;18:427–31.
136. Rasool M, Schuster J, Aslam M, Tariq M, Ahmad I, Ali A, Entesarian M, Dahl N, Baig SM. A novel missense mutation in the EDA gene associated with X-linked recessive isolated hypodontia. J Hum Genet. 2008;53:894–8.
137. Reitan K. Some factors determining the evaluation of forces in orthodontics. Am J Orthod. 1957;43:32–45.
138. Retrouvey J-M, Schwarts S, Hartsfield JK. Oral-facial aspects of osteogenesis imperfecta. In: Shapiro JR, Byers PH, Glorieux FH, Sponseller PD, editors. Osteogenesis imperfecta : a translational approach to brittle bone disease. London: Academic; 2014.
139. Roberts WE, Epker BN, Burr DB, Hartsfield JK, Roberts JA. Remodeling of mineralized tissues, part II: control and pathophysiology. Semin Orthod. 2006;12:238–53. Elsevier.
140. Roberts WE, Roberts JA, Epker BN, Burr DB, Hartsfield JK. Remodeling of mineralized tissues, part I: the frost legacy. Semin Orthod. 2006;12:216–37. Elsevier.
141. Ruf S, Klimas D, Hönemann M, Jabir S. Genetic background of nonsyndromic oligodontia: a systematic review and meta-analysis. J Orofac Orthop. 2013;74:295–308.
142. Sameshima GT, Sinclair PM. Predicting and preventing root resorption: part I. Diagnostic factors. Am J Orthod Dentofacial Orthop. 2001;119:505–10.
143. Sarkar T, Bansal R, Das P. Whole genome sequencing reveals novel non-synonymous mutation in ectodysplasin a (EDA) associated with non-syndromic X-linked dominant congenital tooth agenesis. PLoS One. 2014;9:e106811.
144. Satoh K, Tsutsumi K, Tosa Y, Mikawa M, Hosaka Y. Le Fort III distraction osteogenesis of midface-retrusion in a case of Hajdu Cheny syndrome. J Craniofac Surg. 2002;13:298–302.
145. Schwartz S, Tsipouras P. Oral findings in osteogenesis imperfecta. Oral Surg Oral Med Oral Pathol. 1984;57:161–7.
146. Sharab LY, Morford LA, Dempsey J, Falcão-Alencar G, Mason A, Jacobson E, Kluemper GT, Macri JV, Hartsfield JK. Genetic and treatment-related risk factors associated with external apical root resorption (EARR) concurrent with orthodontia. Orthod Craniofac Res. 2015;18:71–82.
147. Sharpe W, Reed B, Subtelny JD, Polson A. Orthodontic relapse, apical root resorption, and crestal alveolar bone levels. Am J Orthod Dentofacial Orthop. 1987;91:252–8.

148. Sidiropoulou-Chatzigiannis S, Kourtidou M, Tsalikis L. The effect of osteoporosis on periodontal status, alveolar bone and orthodontic tooth movement a literature review. J Int Acad Periodontol. 2007;9:77–84.
149. Smith WK, Steinhauser RA. Vitamin D-resistant rickets with dental abnormalities. Birth Defects Orig Artic Ser. 1971;7:274–5.
150. Song S, Zhao R, He H, Zhang J, Feng H, Lin L. WNT10A variants are associated with non-syndromic tooth agenesis in the general population. Hum Genet. 2014;133:117–24.
151. Stashenko P, Obernesser M, Dewhirst F. Effect of immune cytokines on bone. Immunol Invest. 1989;18:239–49.
152. Stellzig-Eisenhauer A, Decker E, Meyer-Marcotty P, Rau C, Fiebig BS, Kress W, Saar K, Ruschendorf F, Hubner N, Grimm T, Witt E, Weber BH. Primary failure of eruption (PFE) – clinical and molecular genetics analysis. J Orofac Orthop. 2010;71:6–16.
153. Stewart RE, Hollister DW, Rimoin DL. A new variant of Ehlers-Danlos syndrome: an autosomal dominant disorder of fragile skin, abnormal scarring, and generalized periodontitis. Birth Defects Orig Artic Ser. 1977;13:85–93.
154. Stockton DW, Das P, Goldenberg M, D'souza RN, Patel PI. Mutation of PAX9 is associated with oligodontia. Nat Genet. 2000;24:18–9.
155. Suda N, Ogawa T, Kojima T, Saito C, Moriyama K. Non-syndromic oligodontia with a novel mutation of PAX9. J Dent Res. 2011;90:382–6.
156. Suri L, Gagari E, Vastardis H. Delayed tooth eruption: pathogenesis, diagnosis, and treatment. A literature review. Am J Orthod Dentofacial Orthop. 2004;126:432–45.
157. Tao R, Jin B, Guo SZ, Qing W, Feng GY, Brooks DG, Liu L, Xu J, Li T, Yan Y, He L. A novel missense mutation of the EDA gene in a Mongolian family with congenital hypodontia. J Hum Genet. 2006;51:498–502.
158. Tarpey P, Pemberton TJ, Stockton DW, Das P, Ninis V, Edkins S, Andrew Futreal P, Wooster R, Kamath S, Nayak R, Stratton MR, Patel PI. A novel Gln358Glu mutation in ectodysplasin A associated with X-linked dominant incisor hypodontia. Am J Med Genet A. 2007; 143A:390–4.
159. Van Den Boogaard MJ, Creton M, Bronkhorst Y, Van Der Hout A, Hennekam E, Lindhout D, Cune M, Ploos Van Amstel HK. Mutations in *WNT10A* are present in more than half of isolated hypodontia cases. J Med Genet. 2012;49:327–31.
160. Vastardis H, Karimbux N, Guthua SW, Seidman JG, Seidman CE. A human MSX1 homeodomain missense mutation causes selective tooth agenesis. Nat Genet. 1996;13:417–21.
161. Viecilli RF, Katona TR, Chen J, Hartsfield Jr JK, Roberts WE. Orthodontic mechanotransduction and the role of the P2X7 receptor. Am J Orthod Dentofacial Orthop. 2009;135(694):e1–16; discussion 694–5.
162. Vieira AR, D'souza RN, Mues G, Deeley K, Hsin HY, Kuchler EC, Meira R, Patir A, Tannure PN, Lips A, Costa MC, Granjeiro JM, Seymen F, Modesto A. Candidate gene studies in hypodontia suggest role for FGF3. Eur Arch Paediatr Dent. 2013;14:405–10.
163. Vieira AR, Meira R, Modesto A, Murray JC. *MSX1*, *PAX9*, and *TGFA* contribute to tooth agenesis in humans. J Dent Res. 2004;83:723–7.
164. Vieira AR, Modesto A, Meira R, Barbosa ARS, Lidral AC, Murray JC. Interferon regulatory factor 6 (*IRF6*) and fibroblast growth factor receptor 1 (*FGFR1*) contribute to human tooth agenesis. Am J Med Genet A. 2007;143A:538–45.
165. Vieira AR, Seymen F, Patir A, Menezes R. Evidence of linkage disequilibrium between polymorphisms at the *IRF6* locus and isolate tooth agenesis, in a Turkish population. Arch Oral Biol. 2008;53:780–4.
166. Wise GE, Frazier-Bowers S, D'souza RN. Cellular, molecular, and genetic determinants of tooth eruption. Crit Rev Oral Biol Med. 2002;13:323–34.
167. Woolf CM. Missing maxillary lateral incisors: a genetic study. Am J Hum Genet. 1971;23:289–96.
168. Wu FL, Wang LY, Huang YQ, Guo WB, Liu CD, Li SG. Interleukin-1beta +3954 polymorphisms and risk of external apical root resorption in orthodontic treatment: a meta-analysis. Genet Mol Res. 2013;12:4678–86.

169. Xuan K, Jin F, Liu YL, Yuan LT, Wen LY, Yang FS, Wang XJ, Wang GH, Jin Y. Identification of a novel missense mutation of MSX1 gene in Chinese family with autosomal-dominant oligodontia. Arch Oral Biol. 2008;53:773–9.
170. Yamaguchi S, Machida J, Kamamoto M, Kimura M, Shibata A, Tatematsu T, Miyachi H, Higashi Y, Jezewski P, Nakayama A, Shimozato K, Tokita Y. Characterization of novel MSX1 mutations identified in Japanese patients with nonsyndromic tooth agenesis. PLoS One. 2014;9:e102944.
171. Yang Y, Luo L, Xu J, Zhu P, Xue W, Wang J, Li W, Wang M, Cheng K, Liu S, Tang Z, Ring BZ, Su L. Novel EDA p.Ile260Ser mutation linked to non-syndromic hypodontia. J Dent Res. 2013;92:500–6.

Medication Effects on the Rate of Orthodontic Tooth Movement

6

Theodosia N. Bartzela and Jaap C. Maltha

Abstract

In this chapter, we reviewed the effects of medication on bone physiology and orthodontic tooth movement (OTM). The chapter is organized according to the classes of medication, such as synthetic analogues of eicosanoids, analgesics, corticosteroids, insulin, relaxin, as well as calcium and calcium regulators. We looked into well-controlled animal studies because clinical studies were scarce. Topical administration of synthetic analogues of eicosanoids increased the rate of OTM, whereas inhibition of these analogues decreased OTM. Opioid-based analgesics and nonsteroidal anti-inflammatory drugs (NSAIDs) decreased OTM, whereas non-NSAIDs (such as paracetamol) did not affect the rate of OTM. Corticosteroid hormones, calcium and calcium regulators such as exogenous parathyroid hormone (PTH), and thyroxine stimulated OTM in a dose-dependent manner. Treatment with insulin delayed OTM, while relaxin might have a positive effect on relapse, following OTM, because it modulated collagen metabolism. Estrogen supplementation used to overcome postmenopausal problems might slow down OTM, but there was no experimental evidence. Progesterone, bisphosphonates (BP), and local injection of vitamin D_3 delayed OTM. Medications may influence OTM, and for this reason, adequate information on their consumption is essential for orthodontic treatment planning.

T.N. Bartzela, DDS, Dr med dent, MSc, PhD (✉)
Department of Orthodontics, Dentofacial Orthopedics and Pedodontics, Center for Dental and Craniofacial Sciences (CC3), Charité University Clinic,
Aßmannshauser Straße 4-6, Berlin 14197, Germany

Department of Orthodontics, Aristotle University of Thessaloniki, Thessaloniki, Greece
e-mail: theodosia.bartzela@charite.de

J.C. Maltha, PhD
Department of Orthodontics and Craniofacial Biology, Radboud University Nijmegen Medical Centre, 309 Tandheelkunde, Postbus 9101, Nijmegen NL 6500 HB, The Netherlands
e-mail: jaap.maltha@radboudumc.nl

B. Shroff (ed.), *Biology of Orthodontic Tooth Movement*,
DOI 10.1007/978-3-319-26609-1_6

6.1 Introduction

Orthodontists increasingly see patients that use medication for prevention or treatment of various diseases on a regular basis. In the USA, the National Drug Early Warning System (NDEWS) reports data and trends showing that prescription drug abuse explodes. Among prescription medication users, about half used concurrently over-the-counter medications and/or dietary supplements. It is known that medication may have side effects intervening with orthodontic treatment. Orthodontists should be aware of that, as it may result in increase or decrease in the rate of orthodontic tooth movement (OTM) or other unwanted side effects that should be discussed with the patients [15].

Recently, the effects of different types of medication on biological processes related to orthodontic tooth movement have been reviewed [15, 60, 70, 71, 78]. Most of these reviews discuss the possible effects of medication on biological processes related to OTM. Briefly, they conclude that the principal trigger for OTM is probably strain of the periodontal ligament cells, the bone-related cells, and the extracellular matrix. This strain subsequently leads to multiple changes in gene expression in the cells by interactions between cells and extracellular matrix, whereby integrins play an important role. A variety of cell-signaling pathways is activated, which ultimately leads to stimulation of periodontal ligament turnover as well as localized bone resorption and bone deposition. Many of these processes can be modulated by systemic or local application of medications and the intake of dietary supplements, such as vitamins and minerals, suggesting that they may have a stimulatory or inhibitory effect on OTM [28, 32, 61, 111]. In most cases, these authors distinguish two categories of effects: those related to general bone physiology in terms of bone density, bone mineralization, bone turnover rate, and osteoclast differentiation, on one hand, and on the other hand, clinical side effects induced by medications, such as gingival hyperplasia, xerostomia, and external root resorption.

Most reviews, however, have not reported experimental data on the effects of medications or dietary supplements on the rate of OTM itself [11, 33, 89]. Nonetheless, such information is important for clinicians in their communication with their patients, as that many patients use prescription or over-the-counter medications, as well as dietary supplements on a daily basis that it can be considered an "epidemic phenomenon" [46, 61, 111].

High esthetic results and short-lasting treatment are required by many adults seeking orthodontic treatment. Therefore, recently, several systematic reviews have been published about methods that are supposed to possibly accelerate OTM. Although no evidence-based clinical data are available, it is suggested that surgical interventions such as corticotomy and distraction osteogenesis may shorten the orthodontic treatment [44]. Additionally, a systematic review on animal experiments suggests that both corticotomy and distraction osteogenesis lead to an early-stage temporary acceleration of OTM [66]. A systematic review on the clinical effect of low-intensity laser therapy, photobiomodulation, or pulsed electromagnetic fields on the rate of OTM leads only to the suggestion that low-intensity laser therapy may have some effect [34]. These recent reviews indicate an increased interest from the orthodontist to find surgical of physical methods for acceleration of the treatment.

The most recent systematic review on the sequela of pharmaceutical interventions and the use of dietary supplements on the rate of OTM covers the literature up to 2008 [15]. To describe the more recent developments in this field, we performed an update of this review, covering the literature up to June 2015. Unfortunately, only a limited number of clinical trials in humans have been published [90, 105, 119]. Therefore, it has been decided to focus mainly on well-controlled animal studies.

This chapter is organized around several regulatory systems of which disturbances may lead to pathological conditions that affect bone metabolism or give rise to other unwanted signs and symptoms. Most pharmaceutical interventions either aim for an increase in the local production of regulatory factors by stimulating their synthesis or by the administration of synthetic analogues. On the other hand, they often try to counteract the effect of these regulatory factors by selective inhibition of their synthesis or by blocking their active domains.

6.2 Eicosanoids

Eicosanoids are a group of signaling molecules involved in the regulation of a wide variety of regulatory processes and pathological conditions that trigger inflammatory reaction and immune responses, anaphylaxis, vasodilatation and vasoconstriction, coagulation, stimulation of peripheral nerve endings, and the development of (auto)immune diseases.

Four families of eicosanoids can be distinguished: leukotrienes, thromboxanes, prostacyclins, and prostaglandins. All four are derived from arachidonic acid by a variety of enzymatic conversions. Leukotrienes are the only eicosanoids that are converted from arachidonic acid by the action of lipoxygenase and not by cyclooxygenase (COX). All three isoforms of cyclooxygenase (COX), COX-1 COX-2, and COX-3, play a pivotal role for the conversion of arachidonic acid to thromboxanes, prostacyclins, and prostaglandins.

Depending on the pathological condition, the action of eicosanoids may be stimulated by the administration of synthetic analogues or counteracted by direct or indirect inhibitors.

6.2.1 Leukotrienes

Leukotrienes play an important role in inflammation, allergic, and asthmatic reactions. Their effects can be counteracted by antagonists of leukotriene receptors, such as montelukast and zafirlukast, medication used for asthma, or by inhibition of leukotriene synthesis by a drug such as zileuton. Zileuton selectively blocks the essential enzyme lipoxygenase resulting in inhibition of bone resorption, as well as stimulation of bone deposition, thereby possibly influencing OTM [73].

AA861 ((2,3,5-trimethyl-6-(12-hydroxy-5,10-dodecadiynyl)-1,4-benzoquinone)) was used to selectively inhibit the leukotriene synthesis on OTM in a rat model. The first molars were mesialized by force application of 60 cN, and AA861 was administered at a dosage of 20 mg/kg/day. The experimental data showed significant decrease in the rate of OTM [73].

In a more recent study, mice were treated orally with zileuton (30 mg/kg/day) and montelukast (2 mg/kg/day). A force of 35 cN was applied for first molar mesialization. The two experimental groups treated by zileuton and montelukast showed a reduction of 34.5 % and 41 %, respectively, of OTM after 12 days of treatment [74].

These findings suggest that pharmaceuticals such as zileuton, montelukast, and zafirlukast decrease the rate of OTM. Further clinical studies may elucidate whether the same phenomena take place in chronic asthmatic patients under the treatment of antileukotriene drugs [74].

6.2.2 Thromboxanes

Thromboxane A2 (TXA2) is an unstable arachidonic acid metabolite, and thromboxane B2 (TXB2) is an inactive product of TXA2 which stimulates platelet aggregation, atherogenesis, neovascularization, and vasoconstriction. TXA2 is involved in allergic and immune system reactions, while TXB2 is found in increased amounts in the oral cavity in experimental inflammatory conditions (gingivitis and periodontitis). However, no relation with periodontal bone loss could be established [82]. The local administration of the thromboxane analogue U 46619 at dosages between 2.10^{-5} and 2.10^{-3} μM/12 h significantly increased the rate of OTM evoked by a force of 20 cN between rat incisors [37]. This data suggest that inhibition of thromboxane synthesis by, for example, nonsteroidal anti-inflammatory drugs (NSAIDs) (see below) may impede OTM.

6.2.3 Prostacyclins

Prostacyclins (PGI_2), in contrast to thromboxanes, act as vasodilators and prevent platelet aggregation. Synthetic prostacyclin (epoprostenol) or analogues such as iloprost are used for the treatment of ischemic conditions and pulmonary arterial hypertension. However, surprisingly, local iloprost administration at dosages from 2.10^{-5} to 2.10^{-3} μM/12 h significantly increased the rate of OTM evoked by a separation force of 20 cN between rat incisors [37]. This indicates that the effects of prostacyclins and thromboxanes on OTM are comparable, although their effects on platelet aggregation and vasodilatation are contrary. An explanation can be found in in vitro findings showing that stimulation of either thromboxane receptors or prostacyclin receptors leads to an upregulation of COX-2 and subsequently to a positive feedback loop that also includes prostaglandin synthesis [87]. Therefore, the administration of the prostacyclin analogue iloprost as well as the thromboxane analogue U 46619 increases the synthesis of prostaglandins, thereby indirectly stimulating OTM. As for thromboxanes, the synthesis of prostacyclins is inhibited by NSAIDs (see below).

6.2.4 Prostaglandins

Prostaglandins play an important role in inflammation. Furthermore, they have an effect on smooth muscle cells, platelet aggregation, peripheral nerve endings, and calcium homeostasis. Prostaglandins are associated with osteoblastic differentiation [60], increased number of osteoclasts, and new bone formation. Synthetic prostaglandin analogues, such as misoprostol, are used for a variety of conditions, including the prevention of peptic ulcers and the induction of labor.

The effect of exogenous prostaglandins on OTM was studied in monkeys [118]. In a split-mouth design, canine retraction was performed after extraction of the first premolar. The initial force was set at 100 cN, and at one side, local injections of synthetic PGE2 (dinoprostone) were given during a 4-day interval at a dosage of 40 μg. The results suggest faster OTM at the experimental sides, but no statistical analysis was performed [118]. Some other studies in rats are more convincing. In these studies, incisors were separated by a force of 20 cN and 60 cN, respectively. It was shown that the rate of OTM increased significantly in a dose-dependent manner after single or multiple local injections of exogenous prostaglandin (PGE2) at dosages between 0.1 and 10.0 μg [50, 64]. Weekly local injections of 100 μg of exogenous PGE2 also stimulated mesial molar movement in rats induced by a force of 60 cN [93]. Also a study into the effect of administration of an agonist of the prostaglandin receptor EP4, thus stimulating PGE synthesis, on tooth movement in rats showed comparable effects [23].

The effects of exogenous PGE1 (alprostadil) and its synthetic analogue misoprostol on OTM have also been studied. PGE1 stimulates the synthesis and secretion of protective mucus that lines the gastrointestinal tract. Furthermore, it increases mucosal blood flow, thereby improving mucosal integrity. It is sometimes coprescribed with NSAIDs to prevent gastric ulceration, a common adverse effect of NSAIDs.

In an experiment in guinea pigs, a separating force of 25 cN was applied to the incisors [53]. Administration of misoprostol at a dosage of 100 μg/kg/12 h resulted in a significant increase in the rate of tooth separation [53]. The stimulatory effect of misoprostol on incisor separation was also found in a rat study, where misoprostol was administered at different dosages by gastric gavage. A force of 60 cN was used; and dosages of 10 μg/kg/day and more resulted in a significant increase in the rate of OTM [95].

The effect of PGE1 has also been studied in humans and monkeys. The study in monkeys yielded no convincing results due to the lack of statistical analysis [118]. Two investigations in humans using a split-mouth design showed a significant increase in the rate of palatal premolar movement after multiple local injections of PGE1 at a dosage of 10 μg [105, 119].

An indirect way to influence PGE2 synthesis is the use of a diet rich in n-3 polyunsaturated fatty acids. After 5 weeks of feeding such a diet, rats showed lower arachidonic acid and PGE2 concentrations in lipids extracted from the alveolar bone than after a diet rich in n-6 saturated fatty acids [56]. Orthodontic incisor separation with a force of about 56 cN was significantly slower in animals being fed with unsaturated fatty acids diet. Similar results have been shown after buccal movement of maxillary first molars in rats with an initial force of 20 cN [47].

Inhibitors of prostaglandin synthesis have found a widespread application in medicine. NSAIDs represent the most important class of these drugs (see below).

6.3 Analgesic

6.3.1 Nonsteroidal Anti-inflammatory Drugs (NSAIDs)

NSAIDs form the most important class of prostanoid synthesis inhibitors. They have analgesic, antipyretic, and anti-inflammatory effects and are prescribed for a wide variety of conditions, such as rheumatoid arthritis, osteoarthritis, gout, dysmenorrhea, headache, migraine, and (postoperative) pain, as well as for the prevention of cardiovascular diseases and colorectal cancer. The prescriptions show important differences. In case of chronic diseases such as rheumatoid arthritis, osteoarthritis, and gout, relatively high doses are prescribed for a long period of time. For the prevention of cardiovascular problems and colorectal cancer, also long-term prescriptions are given but at a low dose. Finally, for the treatment of, for example, pain and headache, NSAIDs are taken incidentally. This should be considered in evaluating the effects of NSAIDs on OTM.

NSAIDs can be divided into different groups according to their chemical composition. Well-known members of these groups are listed in (Table 6.1).

All NSAIDs have more or less similar effects and mechanisms of action. They suppress the production of all prostanoids (thromboxanes, prostacyclins, and prostaglandins) due to their inhibition of COX-1 and COX-2, which are essential enzymes in the synthetic pathways of the prostanoids. COX-1 is a constitutive form, while COX-2 is inducible. Acetylsalicylic acid, for example, inhibits both types of COX in a noncompetitive and irreversible way [117]; thus, it effectively inhibits prostaglandin synthesis. In the early 1990s, it became apparent [43] that COX-1 mediates the synthesis of prostaglandins responsible for the protection of the stomach lining, while COX-2 is induced during inflammatory reactions, thereby mediating the synthesis of prostaglandins responsible for pain [63, 92].

A special category of NSAIDs are the so-called coxibs. These are specific COX-2 inhibitors developed for the management of osteoarthritis, but they are also used in the therapy of acute or chronic pain and dysmenorrhea. Concerns about the increased risk of cardiac attack and stroke associated with long-term, high-dosage use have in some cases led to either a complete withdrawal from the market (rofecoxib (Vioxx, Ceoxx, and Ceeoxx), valdecoxib (Bextra)) or to a more stringent prescription policy (celecoxib (Celebrex, Celebra)).

Almost all studies on the effects of NSAIDs during experimental OTM in animals evaluate the effects of a relatively short-lasting administration. They have shown a decrease in the number of osteoclasts, since prostaglandins are involved

Table 6.1 Groups and subgroups of NSAIDs and some well-known brand names

NSAIDs	
Salicylates	Aspirin (Aspirin, Acetal, Acetophen, Acetosal, Aspro, and over 100 more) Diflunisal (Dolobid)
Arylalkanoic acids	Diclofenac (Voltaren, Voltarol, Diclon, Dicloflex, Difen, Difene, Cataflam, Pennsaid, Rhumalgan, Abitren) Indometacin (Indocin, Indocid, Indochron) Ketorolac
Arylpropionic acids (profens)	Ibuprofen (Nurofen, Advil, Brufen, Dorival, Panafen, Ibumetin, Ibuprom) Flurbiprofen (ANSAID) Naproxen (Aleve, Anaprox, Naprogesic, Naprosyn, Naprelan)
Oxicams	Piroxicam (Feldene) Meloxicam (Movalis, Melox, Recoxa, Mobic) Tenoxicam (Mobiflex)
Coxibs	Celecoxib (Celebrex, Celebra) Rofecoxib (Vioxx, Ceoxx, Ceeoxx) Valdecoxib (Bextra)

either directly or indirectly in osteoclast differentiation or in stimulating their activity. The effect of NSAIDs on the rate of OTM itself will be discussed for the different groups of NSAIDs separately. This has been shown for acetylsalicylic acid and flurbiprofen [89], indometacin (INN term for the USAN term indomethacin) [33], and ibuprofen [11]. Whether or not this leads to a reduction in the rate of OTM is less clear. There are recommendations that the prostaglandin inhibitors during the orthodontic treatment should be avoided [33]. Acetaminophen was proposed as the analgesic of choice for the orthodontic patients [11].

6.3.1.1 Salicylates

Acetylsalicylic acid is the first discovered and most widely used NSAID.

Acetylsalicylic acid administration in a dosage of 65 mg/kg/day in guinea pigs did not result in a reduction in the rate of lateral incisor movement by mild forces of 8 cN [117]. On the other hand, the rate of lateral incisor movement in rats, evoked by a force of 35 cN, significantly decreased after application of acetylsalicylic acid at a dosage of 100 mg/kg twice a day [11]. However, acetylsalicylic acid administrated at a dose of 60 or 300 mg/kg/day via drinking water did not affect mesial orthodontic tooth movement induced by a force of 50 cN over a period of 14 days [36]. In contrast to this study, molar mesialization was significantly reduced in rats after local injections of 17.5–35 mg/kg/day of Cu salicylate and forces application of 50 or 100 cN for 28 days [54]. The differences in outcome may be related to differences in study design.

6.3.1.2 Arylalkanoic Acids

Administration of a single dose of indometacin (4 mg/kg) in rats resulted in a significant short-lasting inhibitory effect on the mesial movement of molars induced by a force of 40 cN [123]. Other authors employed forces of 60 cN and 50 or 100 cN, respectively, while indometacin was administered at a dosage of 2.5–5 mg/kg/day.

A significant reduction in the rate of molar movement was found during the whole experimental period of 14 and 28 days, respectively, regardless of the force level [54, 73]. The effect of indometacin on OTM has also been studied in cats and miniature pigs. In cats, the third premolars were moved mesially by a force of 250 cN [22]. Using the same application regime for indometacin as in the previously mentioned study, a significant reduction in the rate of OTM was found [22, 73]. In miniature pigs, the incisors were separated by a force of 100 cN. Initially, a dosage of 20 mg/kg/day of indometacin was given, but this had to be changed during the experimental period to 10 mg/kg/day due to peptic ulcer problems [33]. Although no direct tooth movement was measured, the reduced bone turnover strongly suggested a decrease in OTM rate [33].

The effect of diclofenac was studied in a rat model in which mesial tipping of first molars was induced by forces of 50 or 100 cN. Injections of diclofenac (10 mg/kg at day 1 and day 3) abolished OTM completely [27]. These results point in the same direction as a more recent study in rats on the effect of diclofenac. A force of 30 cN was applied on the first molar for 3, 7, or 14 days. Diclofenac was given in a daily dose of 5 mg/kg/day, and after 3 and 7 days, this leads to fewer blood vessels, Howship lacunae, and osteoclast-like cells, suggesting less OTM during the initial phase of treatment [55].

Ketorolac is an analgesic that is used for the short-term relief of moderate to severe pain and should not be used for longer than 5 days and for mild pain or for pain from chronic (long-term) conditions. The only study in which the effect of ketorolac on OTM is studied is in rats, in which a dosage of 3 mg/kg/day was administered by gastric gavage for 2 months. This leads to a decrease in mesial OTM after the application of a force of 50 cN [38]. However, the experimental period is far longer than the prescribed maximal period this drug should be taken, and therefore its clinical relevance is questionable.

6.3.1.3 Arylpropionic Acids

Administration of ibuprofen at an unknown dose for 5 days resulted in a significant reduction of tipping molar movement induced in rats by a mesial force of 50 cN over a period of 21 days [112]. Also, studies in which rat incisors were moved laterally by a force of 25 or 35 cN point in the same direction. After ibuprofen administration at a dose of 30 mg/kg twice a day, the rate of OTM decreased significantly [11]. On the other hand, no inhibitory effect could be found at a low dose (10 mg/kg/day) of flurbiprofen on the mesial movement of rabbit first molars when a force of 100 cN was applied [89].

These clinical studies provide an indirect evaluation of the effect of ibuprofen on the OTM.

Two recent clinical studies that have been performed on the effects of ibuprofen on PGE2 release in the gingival crevicular fluid (GCF), as an indirect indication for their effect on OTM, showed conflicting results. The first evaluated the effect of ibuprofen (400 mg/day for 2 days) during canine distalization with a force of 150 cN. This led to a significant decrease in PGE2 release compared to the control group [97]. In the other study, the participants had taken 400 mg ibuprofen, 1 h before and

6 h after bonding, and GCF samples were taken prior to bonding, after bonding, and 1, 3, and 7 days thereafter. Neither time-related differences nor placebo group differences in PGE2 release was observed [110].

However, OTM is a multifactorial process over a long period of time, and the effect of long-term use of ibuprofen therefore may differ. In patients with chronic illnesses like juvenile rheumatoid arthritis, osteoarthritis, or gout, where long-term analgesic consumption is needed, the inhibiting effects on OTM may become more evident.

6.3.1.4 Oxicams

The effect of meloxicam on OTM was studied in rats in which a force of 50 cN was used to move the maxillary left molar to the mesial for 2 weeks. The animals received a high (67 mg/kg/day)- or low (13 mg/kg/day)-dose meloxicam via their drinking water. No effect on OTM was found over the experimental period [36].

One clinical study also has been performed on the effects of oxicams. In a randomized clinical trial (RCT), bilateral canine retraction was performed over a period of 3 months with monthly reactivation. Tenoxicam (20 mg/day) was given for 3 days around each (re)activation, and the patients had access to additional paracetamol (4 times 750 mg/day). This medication had no effect on OTM [10].

6.3.1.5 Coxibs

The effect of local injections of rofecoxib (1 mg/kg at day 1 and day 3) was studied in a rat model in which mesial movement of the first molar was induced by forces of 50 or 100 cN [27]. It appeared that no OTM occurred when 50 cN were applied, but 100 cN did induce OTM. It was however significantly less than in the controls without medication [27]. In a subsequent study, the same group compared the effects of injections of rofecoxib (0.5 mg/kg), celecoxib (8 mg/kg), or parecoxib (25 mg/kg) on days 0, 3, and 5 after placement of the appliance. OTM was determined after 10 days of treatment. In the rofecoxib-treated animals, no OTM at all was occured, while OTM in the celecoxib and parecoxib treatment was comparable to the controls [27].

In a comparable rat study, in which a longer experimental period was used (14 days), a significant reduction in OTM was found after celecoxib administration [40]. In contrast to these studies, no interference with OTM was found after administration of 50 mg/kg celecoxib by oral gavage, prior to placement of an orthodontic appliance exerting a force of 50 cN. The experimental period was restricted to 48 h of active OTM [106].

A dose-dependent effect of celecoxib in OTM was found in a rat study where doses of 16 mg/kg/day or 3.2 mg/kg/day were administered through the drinking water for 14 days. Only the high dose inhibited OTM [36]. These results are in contrast to a more recent rat study in which celecoxib injections at a low dose (0.3 mg/day) were given every 3 days for a period of 18 days. This resulted in a significant decrease in OTM [102]. However, another recent study, in which daily injections of 10 mg/kg celecoxib was administered in rats for a period of 2 months, could not establish an effect on OTM [38].

6.3.2 Non-NSAID Analgesics

Paracetamol (INN term for the USAN term acetaminophen).

Paracetamol is a very commonly used analgesic. It lacks anti-inflammatory properties. Therefore, it does not belong to the group of NSAIDs, although their chemical structures are comparable. Other important differences are that paracetamol has almost no effect on blood clotting and on the stomach lining. These differences are related to its mode of action. NSAIDs block COX-1 and/or COX-2 and interfere with prostaglandin synthesis, while paracetamol blocks the isoform COX-3 but has no effect on COX-1 or COX-2 nor on PGE2 synthesis [97].

The effect of paracetamol on OTM in rabbits has been studied during administration of a dosage of 500 mg/kg/day. No effect on the rate of mesial molar movement was found when using a force of 100 cN [84]. Likewise, a dosage of 200 mg/kg/day for 2 or 10 days in rats did not influence the rate of lateral displacement of the incisors by applying a force 35 cN [11, 106]. Comparable results were found in a rat study where molars were moved to the mesial by a force of 50 cN, and paracetamol was applied via drinking water at a dose of 20 or 100 mg/kg/day for 2 weeks [36]. However, a recent study showed a significant decrease of OTM in rats where a mesial force of 50 cN was applied for 2 months, and paracetamol was administered by gastric gavage at a dose of 150 mg/kg/day throughout the experimental period [38]. Paracetamol did not affect the rate of OTM with the given dosages, during the 2-week observational period. For this reason, it is suggested that it should be the analgesic of choice for managing pain associated with orthodontic therapy. However, long-term application might result in a decrease in OTM.

6.3.3 Opioids

Opioids are effective for the treatment of acute and chronic-related pain, i.e., with degenerative conditions such as rheumatoid arthritis, or even during labor and cardiac infraction. They work by binding to opioid receptors, which are found principally in the central and peripheral nervous system and the gastrointestinal tract. Only very few studies have been performed on the effects of opioids on OTM. The opioids tested were only morphine (INN) and tramadol (marketed as Ultram and Tramal and as generics). However, tramadol is under strict control in some countries. In one rat study, it is reported that daily morphine injections at a dose of 5 mg/kg/day over 14 days reduced the rate of OTM induced by a force of 60 cN [5]. In another study from the same group, daily tramadol injections at a dose of 20 mg/kg/day during 14 days had no effect [81]. These results are supported by a rat study in which again a force of 60 cN was used to move rat molars to the mesial for 14 days. Administration of tramadol at 10 mg/kg/day had no significant effect on OTM, while after administration of increasing doses up to 60 mg/kg/day, OTM almost completely came to a standstill [4].

6.4 Corticosteroids

Corticosteroids form a class of steroid hormones, produced in the adrenal cortex. Some corticosteroids, the glucocorticoids (cortisone, cortisol, prednisolone, and methylprednisolone) are involved in the control of carbohydrate, fat, and protein metabolism. They are also participated in bone physiology, but their mode of action is not yet completely elucidated. Osteoblasts and osteoclasts can express glucocorticoid receptors under the influence of pro-inflammatory factors, such as IL-6 and IL-11. Glucocorticoids are prescribed for a variety of inflammatory and (auto)immune conditions, including rheumatoid arthritis, dermatitis, allergies, and asthma. They are also used as immunosuppressive medications after organ transplantation. Their anti-inflammatory function is based on the indirect blocking of phospholipase A2 and the suppression of the synthesis of both COX-1 and COX-2. This leads to an inhibition of the synthesis of prostaglandins and leukotrienes. Their immunosuppressive action is due to the inhibition of interleukins and IFN-γ. Other corticosteroids (mineralocorticoids), such as aldosterone, control mainly electrolyte and water levels by promoting sodium retention in the kidneys.

6.4.1 Glucocorticoids

6.4.1.1 Cortisone

The effect of cortisone on OTM was investigated in rabbits. Cortisone acetate was injected at a dosage of 15 mg/kg/day for 4 days before, as well as during the application of an orthodontic force of approximately 100 cN for a period of 14 days. Compared to controls, this regime led to a significant increase in the rate of OTM. Also, the relapse rate was faster in the experimental than in the control animals [13].

6.4.1.2 Prednisolone

In a rat study was tested the effect of two dosages of prednisolone (0.13 and 0.67 mg/kg/day) administered through the drinking water over a period of 14 days. It showed a dose-dependent suppression of OTM [36]. In another study, prednisolone was administered at 1 mg/kg/day in rats for an induction period of 12 days, followed by a subsequent experimental period of 12 days. During the latter phase of the study, the first molar was moved mesially with a force of 30 cN. This therapy had no significant effect on the rate of OTM [77].

6.4.1.3 Methylprednisolone

In one of the experimental groups, an induction period of 7 weeks was used, whereupon OTM was performed for 3 weeks with a force of 25 cN in which methylprednisolone was given at a dosage of 8 mg/kg/day [51]. This led to an increase in the rate of OTM. However, in another experimental group where the induction period was omitted, methylprednisolone had no effect on the rate of OTM [51].

6.4.2 Mineralocorticoids

No experimental study was found dealing with mineralocorticoids.

6.4.3 Triamcinolone

Triamcinolone is a synthetic corticosteroid. It is used to treat various ophthalmologic and skin conditions or to relieve mouth sores. The derivative triamcinolone acetonide is one of the ingredients of Ledermix, used during root canal treatment. The effect of triamcinolone acetonide on OTM has recently been studied in rabbits. The drug was injected at a dose of 1 mg/kg/day for 21 days, and the incisors were moved by a force of 50 cN for the same period. A significant increase in OTM was found [1]. The differences in the results of the studies on glucocorticoids probably reflect the combined effects of the applied dosages, the induction periods, and the relative anti-inflammatory activity of the glucocorticoids tested.

6.5 Insulin/Relaxin

6.5.1 Insulin

The human insulin is a peptide hormone produced by beta cells in the pancreas. It regulates the metabolism of carbohydrates and fats by promoting the absorption of glucose from the blood to skeletal muscles and fat tissue. It also inhibits the production of glucose by the liver. When control of insulin levels fails, diabetes mellitus can result. As a consequence, insulin is used medically to treat some forms of diabetes mellitus (type 1 diabetes, injected subcutaneously). Patients with type 2 diabetes are often insulin resistant and may eventually require insulin if dietary modifications or other medications fail to control blood glucose levels. In only one study, the effect of insulin treatment in mice with induced diabetes type 1 on OTM is measured. Diabetes was induced by weekly intraperitoneal injections of 120 mg/kg of streptozotocin. Another group was treated with insulin after diabetes induction. Tooth movement was evoked by a mesial force of 35 cN. OTM in the diabetic animals was faster than in the controls. Treatment with insulin resulted in slower OTM than in the normal animals [17]. One other study was performed in rats with a comparable experimental design. However, in this study, OTM itself was not measured, but the presented histomorphometric data point in the same direction: increase in bone remodeling in diabetic animals and return to about normal values after insulin treatment [115].

6.5.2 Relaxin

Relaxin belongs to the insulin superfamily, and it is an ovarian hormone that stimulates osteoclastic and osteoblastic activities and connective tissue turnover. In humans it is produced in males and in both pregnant and nonpregnant women. In addition, relaxin is a potent vasodilator with a number of pleiotropic effects. In recent years, scientific interest has been raised with respect to relaxin as a compound for use in the management of acute heart failure (AHF) [116]. It has also been proposed as a pharmacological agent for the treatment of primary varicosis (chronic venous insufficiency, CVI) which is a widely prevailing venous disease [3]. Relaxin can reduce the level of PDL organization and increase tooth mobility, in the early time of experimental evaluation, but not the OTM [69]. These were the results of mesially evoked force of 40 cN in rats which had previously received relaxin or vehicle treatments for 1 or 3 days [69]. In another experimental design, only the relapse after the completion of OTM was evaluated in rat molars. It was concluded that because relaxin modulates the collagen metabolism, it may be effective for the relapse following OTM [42].

6.6 Calcium and Calcium Regulators

Calcium is essential in a variety of physiological processes, for example, muscle contraction, fluid balance, heartbeat, and enzyme regulation. An important aspect of calcium metabolism is plasma calcium homeostasis. When the blood plasma calcium level in humans rises above its set point, calcitonin is released by the thyroid gland, and the plasma calcium level returns to normal. If on the other hand, calcium falls below that set point, parathyroid hormone (PTH) is released by the parathyroid glands in order to keep the plasma calcium homeostasis. Hormones, such as thyroid hormones (thyroxine, calcitonin) and sex hormones (estrogens), as well as vitamins (e.g., vitamin D_3) and dietary intake of calcium are important regulators of calcium homeostasis. They control the expression and secretion of receptor activator of nuclear factor κB ligand (RANKL) and osteoprotegerin (OPG). RANKL is a cytosine secreted by bone marrow cells, osteoblasts, and osteocytes, and it plays an important role in osteoclast generation [86]. RANK is the receptor for RANKL on the osteoclast precursors and part of the RANK/RANKL/OPG-signaling pathway. The binding of RANKL to RANK stimulates the osteoclast differentiation, and consequently, it stimulates bone resorption. OPG is a soluble decoy-RANK receptor. If it binds to RANKL, it inhibits the interaction between RANKL and RANK, thus suppressing osteoclast differentiation. Consequently, skeletal homeostasis involves interactions between systemic hormones and the local RANKL/RANK/OPG system [86]. A separate class of drugs that affect calcium homeostasis are the bisphosphonates.

6.6.1 Parathyroid Hormone (PTH)

Parathyroid hormone (PTH) consists of 84 amino acids, but the active fragment contains only the amino acids 1–34. Its main effect is an increase in the concentration of calcium in the blood. PTH binds to osteoblasts, stimulating the expression of RANKL.

Pathological PTH conditions might involve hypoparathyroidism and hyperparathyroidism. Hypoparathyroidism leads to a shortage of active PTH. There is no direct way of influencing thyroid hormone secretion by the thyroid gland. The most widely used therapy is the exogenous vitamin D and/or calcium (see below) or/and a synthetic long-acting form of thyroxine, known as levothyroxine (L-thyroxine).

In primary hyperparathyroidism, overproduction of the hormone stimulates bone resorption, reduces renal clearance of calcium, and increases intestinal calcium absorption, which results in increased serum calcium levels. The therapy involves medication with bisphosphonates (see below) or even surgical removal of the glands. In secondary hyperparathyroidism, the secretion of PTH is increased due to hypocalcemia. The treatment consists of vitamin D_3 supplementation (see below) or the use of phosphate binders.

Although short and intermittent elevations of the PTH level can be anabolic for the bone, the continuous elevation of the hormone induces bone loss [80]. The only bone growing anabolic agent is teriparatide. It is a recombinant form of the active (1–34) fragment of PTH. The intermittent use of teriparatide activates osteoblasts more than osteoclasts, and therefore, it is used for the treatment of advanced osteoporosis [85]. Daily injections of teriparatide promote new bone formation and increase bone mineral density [48]. Also in ovariectomized animals, teriparatide administration at a dose of 30 mug/kg/day for 90 days has stimulated OTM 1 week after the force application [88].

Exogenous administration of PTH was studied in rats [103, 104]. The rate of OTM was significantly increased in a dose-dependent manner and only when PTH was applied rather continuously, either by systemic infusion [103] or by local, slow release every other day [104]. Total (1–84) PTH was as effective as the (1–34) fragment, in dosages ranged from 0.1 to 1.0 μg/kg/day. If PTH was administered in intermittent short-lasting applications, OTM was not significantly accelerated. This was probably because osteoblastic activity was stimulated, but osteoclastic activity was not affected [104]. However, in a comparable experimental design in male Wistar rats, short-term injection of PTH at a dose of 0.4 μg/kg/day increased bone turnover rate and subsequently OTM [65].

Indirect evidence for the effect of PTH on the rate of OTM may be derived from studies dealing with low-calcium diet, resulting in increased PTH release (see below) [35, 72].

6.6.2 Thyroid Hormones

The thyroid gland produces two hormones, thyroxine and calcitonin.

6.6.2.1 Thyroxine

Thyroxine (T4) is a prohormone that can be converted to its active form triiodothyronine (T3). T4 affects intestinal calcium absorption; as such it is indirectly involved in bone turnover. T3, the active hormone, increases the rate of cell metabolism, and it plays an important role in physical growth, body temperature, and heart rate. Hyperthyroidism or thyroxine medication may lead to osteoporosis.

The effect of exogenous thyroxine on OTM has been studied in a rat model. After an induction period of 4 weeks, 0.003 % thyroxine was added to the drinking water of the animals. Orthodontic force of 25 cN was applied on the first molar for 21 days. Exogenous thyroid hormone increases the rate of OTM in rats [114]. Intraperitoneal administration of thyroxin in dosages of 5, 10, and 20/mg/kg/day resulted in a dose-dependent acceleration of OTM evoked by a force application of 60 cN [99]. More recently, this effect of thyroxine application was confirmed in an experiment with rats after injection of thyroxine at a dose of 20 μg/kg [94].

6.6.2.2 Calcitonin

Calcitonin (CT) has the opposite effects of PTH. It decreases intestinal calcium absorption, osteoclast activity in bone, and renal calcium reabsorption. It is used for the treatment of postmenopausal osteoporosis, hypocalcaemia, and Paget's disease. CT is sometimes used for pain relief after vertebral fracture [86].

Although CT is involved in bone remodeling and calcium homeostasis, no experimental data is available on the effect of exogenous CT application on the rate of OTM. The CT level was evaluated in both tension and compression sites in GCF of upper central incisors in children. Increased level of CT was detected after 24 h to 15 days in the compression site of the teeth, suggesting a stimulatory effect of CT on OTM. CT values were negatively associated with patients' pain perception [6].

6.6.3 Estrogens

Estrogens are female sex hormones that occur naturally in three forms. The first form is estradiol, which regulates the reproductive female cycles. The second form is estrone, which is produced after menopause. The third form, estriol, is expressed primarily during pregnancy. Estrogen supplementation has been used to overcome postmenopausal problems. However, this treatment was related with increased risk of breast cancer, strokes, and other cardiac problems. The development of selective estrogen receptor modulators (SERMs) such as raloxifene is able to minimize the adverse effects of estrogens. Although SERMs improve bone mineral density (BMD) in osteoporotic patients, they do not completely rule out the risks. They reduce the risk of breast and endometrial cancer but not the risk of death from venous thromboembolic events (VTE) and stroke. Therefore, a careful risk–benefit analysis is essential prior to its use in osteoporotic patients [31].

No experimental studies are available in which exogenous estrogens or raloxifene has been administered for an evaluation of their effect on OTM. All available studies evaluate the indirect effect of estrogens on OTM. One study has focused at the rate of buccal movement of molars evoked by a force of 12.5 cN in the course of the normal estrous cycle in rats. It was found that the rate of OTM was inversely related to the estrogen serum level [39]. Another study has looked into the effect of ovariectomy (OVX) on buccal movement of rat molars evoked by a force of 10 cN. A significant increase in the rate of OTM has been established [121]. These results are in agreement with more recent rat studies in which OTM was induced 4 or 8 weeks after

OVX [12, 100, 101] and a study in cats were OTM was significantly slower in the estrous cats than in OVX or anestrous animals [19]. Some authors suggest that estrogen supplementation and raloxifene may slow down OTM, but again, no experimental evidence is available.

6.6.4 Progesterone

Progesterone (P4) and estradiol (E2) are ovarian steroid hormones and play a substantial role in the female reproductive function. E2 has a crucial effect on epiphyseal bone closure. Derivative of E2 is the ethinyl estradiol (EE2), which is used as oral contraceptive. Another hormonal contraceptive is a synthetic progesterone called norgestrel. Hormonal contraceptives induce a reduction of estrogen and a suppression of endogenous progesterone. The use of these contraceptives is associated with endometrial hyperplasia or endometrial cancer. For eliminating these risk factors, hormonal contraceptives are generally prescribed with progesterone. Only few experimental studies are available on this topic. In a rat study, an oral contraceptive consisting of 100 μg/kg/day of ethinyl estradiol plus 1 mg/kg/day of norgestrel was administered 1 week prior to appliance insertion and during the orthodontically induced tooth movement. Maxillary central incisors were moved distally by a force application of 30 cN. Two weeks after the force application, the OTM was significantly slower in the experimental group. This leads to the conclusion that oral contraceptives can significantly inhibit OTM [76]. These results are in agreement with a rabbit study in which long-term progesterone administration reduced experimental OTM [79].

6.6.5 1, 25-Dihydroxycholecalciferol (Vitamin D_3)

1,25(OH)2D (now known as the D hormone) has multiple biologic effects.

Vitamin D (cholecalciferol) is a pleiotropic steroid hormone and is the prohormone of 1,25-dihydroxycholecalciferol ($1,25(OH)_2D_3$). Vitamin D is rarely found in food as D_3 in animal sources and as D_2 in vegetal sources. It regulates calcium and phosphate serum levels by promoting their intestinal absorption and reabsorption in the kidney. Vitamin D deficiency is also associated with periodontal disease, rickets, and osteomalacia as well as other autoimmune, cardiovascular, and metabolic disorders [24]. Therapy for $1,25(OH)_2D_3$ deficiency involves dietary changes or taking $1,25(OH)_2D_3$ supplementation. Active vitamin D compounds are used against osteoporosis. Hypervitaminosis D causes hypocalcemia and may lead to conditions such as anorexia, nausea, polyuria, and eventually renal failure. It can be treated with a low-calcium diet and corticosteroids. Several animal studies are available on the effect of topical injections of $1,25(OH)_2D_3$ on OTM. The studies vary largely in the application regimes. Repeated injections are given in all studies, but the dosages vary. Injections of 10-100 pg/ml showed a dose-dependent increase in OTM in cats [25]. A study in young and adult rats used 20 μl 10^{-10} or 10^{-8} mol/l in the young animals, which leads to a significant dose-dependent increase in OTM, while the same regime in adult animals showed more increase in OTM with the lowest dose (20 μl 10^{-10} mol/l) than with the higher dose (10^{-8} mol/l) [109]. Also another rat study showed a stimulation of OTM after repeated injections with 20 μl 10^{-10} mol/l vitamin D_3 [50]. Normal physiological doses of 1,25(OH)2D_3 in humans are in the order of 20–30 ng/ml. It is well establish that, small variation within the physiological range may affect bone resorption [107] and thus OTM.

6.6.6 Dietary Calcium

Dietary recommendations for calcium intake for children aged 4–8 years is 800 mg/day and for adults between 1000 and 1300 mg/day [99]. Normally, the net absorption from the diet is only 500 mg/day. Calcium supplementation is often prescribed for the prevention of osteoporosis in postmenopausal women. However, increased dietary calcium intake is related to cardiovascular risk events, and therefore, the routine use of calcium supplements has been questioned. The effect of dietary calcium on OTM has been studied in dogs. The animals were fed low- or high-calcium diets for a period of 10 weeks. Eight weeks after premolar extraction, orthodontic force of 100 cN induced in the low-calcium regime led to a significantly higher rate of OTM than the high-calcium diet [72]. These results are in agreement with a comparable study in rats, in which lactating animals were fed a low-calcium diet for 1 week prior to orthodontic force application. OTM induced by a force of 60 cN was higher than in the control animals [35]. These results were probably the result of the quick response of trabecular bone to low-calcium feeding. Low calcium led to an increase in PTH release, thus stimulating bone remodeling [96].

6.6.7 Bisphosphonates

Bisphosphonates can be broadly classified into the non-nitrogen-containing (e.g., clodronate, tiludronate, and etidronate) and the nitrogen-containing BPs (N-BPs, e.g., pamidronate, alendronate, ibandronate, risedronate, and zoledronate). They are used primarily for the prevention and therapy of osteoporosis, Paget's disease, bone metastases, and bone pain from some types of cancer [16, 29, 58, 59, 121]. The mode of action differs between both groups, but the final outcome is the same. They build in the extracellular bone matrix and inhibit bone resorption. Once built in, bisphosphonates have extremely long half-life of 10 years or more. They can again be released as an active drug during normal bone metabolism. Therefore, they may affect bone metabolism for many years after the patient has completed therapy [121]. Bisphosphonate-related osteonecrosis of the jaws (BRONJ) is a complication described in the long-term bisphosphonate treatment [7, 8, 16, 26, 75]. This is caused by the suppressive and anti-angiogenic effects on epithelial cells and inhibitory effect on endothelial cell proliferation [8] and wound healing [18, 62]. The relatively high prevalence of BPONJ in the jaws and specifically in the mandible is mainly due to the fact that the alveolar bone has approximately 10 times more bone turnover than other bones; thus, the accumulation and release of bisphosphonates in alveolar bone is significantly higher [30]. Furthermore, the mandible contains a large amount of cortical bone, whereas the maxilla contains more marrow, and thus the microcirculation is more extensive [83].

Most early experimental research on the effect of bisphosphonates on the rate of OTM has been performed by the Mitani group [2, 45, 67]. A similar model and protocol were used consistently throughout their experiments. They induced lateral or mesial movement in rat molars with a force of approximately 15 cN. A considerable number of studies have been published in which topical or systemic administration of bisphosphonates resulted in a dose-dependent decrease in the rate of OTM. This has been shown in mice [30], rats [21, 41, 49, 52], and rabbits [113]. Only few studies have been performed in orthodontic patients. They comprise case reports, case series, and retrospective cohort studies [57, 68, 83, 122]. They are rather uniform in their conclusions, namely, the orthodontic tooth movement under bisphosphonate medication is possible, especially in low-risk patients (low dose and short period of intake). The final outcome of orthodontic treatment in these patients showed longer treatment duration, incomplete space closure, poor root parallelism, poor incisor alignment, sclerotic areas, and wide PDL with tooth mobility in some cases. Therefore, the altered bone metabolism and higher extent of side effects should be considered in treatment planning, especially in extraction cases or high-risk patients. On the other hand, bisphosphonate therapy might be beneficial for orthodontic anchorage control, skeletal relapse after maxillary expansion or mandibular distraction and similar procedures. Further long-term prospective randomized controlled trials are required to assess possible benefits and adverse effects of bisphosphonate treatment, before bisphosphonates can be therapeutically used in orthodontics.

A complicating factor is the increasing off-label use of bisphosphonates in children [108] for the treatment of primary osteoporosis in conditions like osteogenesis imperfecta and Ehlers–Danlos or Marfan syndrome or even for the treatment of secondary osteoporosis associated with cerebral palsy, cystic fibrosis, anorexia nervosa, idiopathic juvenile arthritis, diabetes mellitus, and childhood cancer. The use of bisphosphonate therapy in pediatric patients remains controversial because of inadequate long-term efficacy and safety data. Therefore, limiting the use of bisphosphonates to those children with recurrent extremity fractures, symptomatic vertebral collapse, and reduced bone mass is advocated. More research is needed to define appropriate indications for bisphosphonate therapy in pediatric patients and the optimal agent, dose, and duration of use [14].

6.7 Discussion and Conclusions

Clinicians become more and more focused on methods for acceleration of the orthodontic treatment because increasing numbers of patients of all ages are seeking orthodontic treatment with an increased demand for optimal result in the shortest treatment duration possible [34, 44]. Orthodontists are very often confronted with patients that use medications on a regular basis, as prescription and/or over-the-counter drug use is ever expanding in advanced societies. For example, the average American citizen receives more than 10 prescriptions per year. The overall medication consumption has been increased because the number of first-time users has increased, more current users take their medications for a longer period of time, and more individuals take more than one medication at the same time [9]. This chapter focuses on data related to the effect of medication on the rate of orthodontic tooth movement. It comprises almost exclusively experimental animal studies, as designed prospective clinical trials are scarce. Comparison of the data from the included studies is hampered by the large variability in experimental design, animal models, administration regimes, and force characteristics. Another problem is that direct extrapolation of experimental animal studies to the clinical situation is not well possible. However, the effects of medication point most likely in the same direction in the experimental animal studies as in the clinical situation. The most frequently prescribed classes of medications, such as antidepressants, anti-ulcerants, cholesterol reducers, and broad-spectrum antibiotics, may be involved in orthodontically undesired side effects [61], but no effect on the rate of OTM has been identified from the use of these medications. Therefore, these medication classes have not been addressed in this chapter.

Topical administration of synthetic analogues of eicosanoids increases the rate of OTM, while their inhibitors may decrease it. The most important inhibitors are the NSAIDs, which have both an analgesic and an anti-inflammatory effect. Although they all show a comparable action pathway, their effect on the rate of OTM is not uniform. It should be realized that the studies on the effects of NSAIDs on OTM are all performed over a relatively short experimental period. The effects found in these studies, therefore, cannot estimate the effects of the prolonged use of the medication in patients with rheumatoid arthritis or with increased risk of cardiovascular diseases including the various side effects listed (risk of adverse cardiovascular reactions or gastrointestinal bleeding events).

From the non-NSAID analgesics, only paracetamol has been studied in relation to orthodontics, and no effect on the rate of OTM could be established. However, serious skin reactions and liver damage have been reported. Therefore, orthodontists should educate themselves in finding safe analgesics that do not interfere with the orthodontic treatment, depending on the individual medical record of their patients.

Opioid-based analgesics reduce OTM in rats [4, 5]. This effect was reversed by the morphine antagonist naltrexone [5].

Corticosteroids, and especially glucocorticoids, stimulate OTM, but this is dependent on the relative anti-inflammatory activity of the corticosteroid used and the administration protocol. Local or systemic application of PTH also increases the rate of OTM. The same effect is seen, if endogenous PTH synthesis is stimulated by, for example, a low-calcium diet. Intermittent short administration of PTH or its active 1–34 fragment (teriparatide), on the other hand, has an anabolic effect on the bone. However, no data has been found showing that such an administration regime inhibits OTM [48]. Administration of exogenous thyroxine increases the rate of OTM in a dose-dependent manner [99, 114]. Although calcitonin (CT) is involved in bone remodeling and calcium homeostasis, no experimental data is available, on its effect on the rate of OTM. CT has been negatively associated with the perception of pain in initial orthodontic tooth movement in young patients [6].

Estrogen supplementation, and specific estrogen receptor modulators (such as raloxifene), may have an inverse relation on the induced OTM. However, data showing a direct effect of estrogen on OTM has not been found in literature.

A case report on a postmenopausal orthodontic patient suggested that the estrogens used for the treatment of osteoporosis may have delayed the OTM, and they may have inhibited alveolar bone loss in the patient's chronic periodontitis [91].

Progesterone in long-term administration and oral contraceptives (ethinyl estradiol and norgestrel, prescribed together) could reduce the rate of OTM [76, 79].

Administration of vitamin D_3 increases the rate of OTM in a dose-dependent manner by frequent application, which is rather impractical if we want to apply it in the orthodontic clinic. The systemic administration of vitamin D has also been under consideration, but long-term safety data is lacking [24]. Often, the systemic administration of vitamin D is combined with calcium. In this case, we cannot draw conclusions about their effect on OTM if vitamin D or calcium has been examined as monotherapies and not as combined supplementation. Their combined use, though, is under safety consideration in terms of cardiovascular events [20].

Dietary calcium in low dose resulted in an increased rate of OTM in comparison to the high-calcium regime [35, 72, 96]. Calcium supplementation is often prescribed for the prevention of osteoporosis in postmenopausal women. Increased doses of dietary calcium have been related to cardiovascular risk events.

Bisphosphonate administration decreases the rate of OTM in a dose-dependent manner. The use of bisphosphonates can lead to complications due to serious osteonecrosis in the maxilla and mandible [121]. This threat is largest in patients which are on prolonged use and intravenous bisphosphonate therapy. Due to the extremely long half-life of these drugs, patients can experience problems even years after they have discontinued therapy. The dental clinician needs to be aware of the potential risk of bisphosphonate-related necrosis of the jaws (BRONJ) in these patients. The reported incidence rate of osteonecrosis is 1:5000 after 2–3 years of discontinuation of BP treatment [122]. Treatment of osteoporosis with teriparatide is a good alternative for patients undergoing orthodontic treatment [88]. However, teriparatide can cause serious side effects, such as decrease in blood pressure or increase plasma calcium level.

Only a few case reports and one retrospective cohort study on orthodontic patient treated with BP are available [59, 68, 83, 122].

In patients with low dose and short period of bisphosphonate intake, orthodontic treatment is possible. In these patients, orthodontic treatment with light force application, frequent monitoring and avoidance of extractions has been recommended. In one case, a complete cessation of OTM has been reported as a side effect of the treatment [83]. Additional side effects are incomplete space closure and poor root parallelism. In high-risk patients, the orthodontic treatment is unpredictable.

It has been suggested that in orthodontic patients, bisphosphonates can be used to prevent relapse, but great caution should be applied [121].

In conclusion, this chapter has shown that experimental evidence for the effects of many prescription and over-the-counter drug medications on OTM is still lacking. The rate of OTM and the medication consumed by the orthodontic patients apparently has not been considered to be an issue for many years.

As mentioned above, medications are also increasingly prescribed to children and adolescents these days. Consequently, orthodontists should assume that many of their patients are taking prescription or over-the-counter medications on a regular basis [46]. This requires that the orthodontist should identify these patients by carefully questioning them about their medication history as well as their consumption of food supplements. We recommend that such an inquiry be a part of every orthodontic diagnosis. Our role as orthodontists is not only to treat the malocclusion but also to identify the biochemical profile of each patient down to the molecular interaction level. We have to be aware of medical considerations of each patient and relate them with possible implications with our treatment.

Furthermore there is a need for more well-designed experimental studies on the effects of different medications on OTM. For the clinician, it is important to translate the animal experimental data into clinical information. In the available, reviewed literature are only isolated clinical orthodontic case reports, which hamper this process.

The use of patients in clinical trials with a systemic use of a drug for acceleration of OTM may present a severe ethical dilemma. For the same reason, local drug administration is sometimes impractical.

It still remains essential that more evidence should be gathered to guide the orthodontist, and further investigations are needed to fill knowledge gaps.

6.8 Appendix

6.8.1 Websites

General information on the medications and their effects on different mediators as presented in this review is mainly web-based information derived from the following sites:

http://en.wikipedia.org; www.nlm.nih.gov/medlineplus; www.rxlist.com; www.drugs.com

http://www.fda.gov/References to these websites are omitted in the following text.

References

1. Abtahi M, Shafaee H, Saghravania N, et al. Effect of corticosteroids on orthodontic tooth movement in a rabbit model. J Clin Pediatr Dent. 2014;38:285–9.
2. Adachi H, Igarashi K, Mitani H, et al. Effects of topical administration of a bisphosphonate (risedronate) on orthodontic tooth movements in rats. J Dent Res. 1994;73:1478–86.
3. Adams J, Schott S, Bern A, et al. A novel role for relaxin-2 in the pathogenesis of primary varicosis. PLoS One. 2012;7:e39021.
4. Aghili H, Moghadam MG, Yassaei S, et al. Effect of tramadol at different doses on orthodontic tooth movement and bone resorption in rats. Dent Res J (Isfahan). 2013;10:337–42.
5. Akhoundi MS, Dehpour AR, Rashidpour M, et al. The effect of morphine on orthodontic tooth movement in rats. Aust Orthod J. 2010;26:113–8.
6. Alarcon JA, Linde D, Barbieri G, et al. Calcitonin gingival crevicular fluid levels and pain discomfort during early orthodontic tooth movement in young patients. Arch Oral Biol. 2013;58:590–5.
7. Allegra A, Oteri G, Alonci A, et al. Association of osteonecrosis of the jaws and POEMS syndrome in a patient assuming rituximab. J Craniomaxillofacial Surg. 2014;42:279–82.
8. Allegra A, Oteri G, Nastro E, et al. Patients with bisphosphonates-associated osteonecrosis of the jaw have reduced circulating endothelial cells. Hematol Oncol. 2007;25:164–9.
9. Anonymous National Institute for Health Care Management. Prescription drug expenditures in 2001: another year of escalating costs. Revised 6 May 2002. www.nihcm.org. 28 Jan 2008.
10. Arantes GM, Arantes VM, Ashmawi HA, et al. Tenoxicam controls pain without altering orthodontic movement of maxillary canines. Orthod Craniofac Res. 2009;12:14–9.
11. Arias OR, Marquez-Orozco MC. Aspirin, acetaminophen, and ibuprofen: their effects on orthodontic tooth movement. Am J Orthod Dentofacial Orthop. 2006;130:364–70.
12. Arslan SG, Arslan H, Ketani A, et al. Effects of estrogen deficiency on tooth movement after force application: an experimental study in ovariectomized rats. Acta Odontol Scand. 2007;65:319–23.
13. Ashcraft MB, Southard KA, Tolley EA. The effect of corticosteroid-induced osteoporosis on orthodontic tooth movement. Am J Orthod Dentofacial Orthop. 1992;102:310–9.
14. Bachrach LK, Ward LM. Clinical review 1: bisphosphonate use in childhood osteoporosis. J Clin Endocrinol Metab. 2009;94:400–9.
15. Bartzela T, Turp JC, Motschall E, et al. Medication effects on the rate of orthodontic tooth movement: a systematic literature review. Am J Orthod Dentofacial Orthop. 2009;135:16–26.
16. Bhatt RN, Hibbert SA, Munns CF. The use of bisphosphonates in children: review of the literature and guidelines for dental management. Aust Dent J. 2014;59:9–19.
17. Braga SM, Taddei SR, Andrade Jr I, et al. Effect of diabetes on orthodontic tooth movement in a mouse model. Eur J Oral Sci. 2011;119:7–14.
18. Braga SM, Taddei SR, Andrade Jr I, et al. Effect of diabetes on orthodontic tooth movement in a mouse model. The effect of morphine on orthodontic tooth movement in rats. Bisphosphonate effects on the behaviour of oral epithelial cells and oral fibroblasts. Effect of alendronate on orthodontic tooth movement in rats. Eur J Oral Sci. 2009;119:7–14.
19. Celebi AA, Demirer S, Catalbas B, et al. Effect of ovarian activity on orthodontic tooth movement and gingival crevicular fluid levels of interleukin-1beta and prostaglandin E(2) in cats. Angle Orthod. 2013;83:70–5.
20. Challoumas D, Stavrou A, Pericleous A, et al. Effects of combined vitamin D – calcium supplements on the cardiovascular system: should we be cautious? Atherosclerosis. 2015;238:388–98.
21. Choi J, Baek SH, Lee JI, et al. Effects of clodronate on early alveolar bone remodeling and root resorption related to orthodontic forces: a histomorphometric analysis. Am J Orthod Dentofacial Orthop. 2010;138:548 e541–548; discussion 548–9.
22. Chumbley AB, Tuncay OC. The effect of indomethacin (an aspirin-like drug) on the rate of orthodontic tooth movement. Am J Orthod. 1986;89:312–4.

23. Chung CJ, Baik HS, Soma K. Bone formation and tooth movement are synergistically enhanced by administration of EP4 agonist. Am J Orthod Dentofacial Orthop. 2007;132:427 e413–420.
24. Cianferotti L, Marcocci C. Subclinical vitamin D deficiency. Best Pract Res Clin Endocrinol Metab. 2012;26:523–37.
25. Collins MK, Sinclair PM. The local use of vitamin D to increase the rate of orthodontic tooth movement. Am J Orthod Dentofacial Orthop. 1988;94:278–84.
26. Consolaro A. The use of bisphosphonates does not contraindicate orthodontic and other types of treatment! Dental Press J Orthod. 2014;19:18–26.
27. De Carlos F, Cobo J, Diaz-Esnal B, et al. Orthodontic tooth movement after inhibition of cyclooxygenase-2. Am J Orthod Dentofacial Orthop. 2006;129:402–6.
28. Diravidamani K, Sivalingam SK, Agarwal V. Drugs influencing orthodontic tooth movement: an overall review. J Pharm Bioallied Sci. 2012;4:S299–303.
29. Fleisch H. Development of bisphosphonates. Breast Cancer Res. 2002;4:30–4.
30. Fujimura Y, Kitaura H, Yoshimatsu M, et al. Influence of bisphosphonates on orthodontic tooth movement in mice. Eur J Orthod. 2009;31:572–7.
31. Fujiwara S, Hamaya E, Sato M, et al. Systematic review of raloxifene in postmenopausal Japanese women with osteoporosis or low bone mass (osteopenia). Clin Interv Aging. 2014;9:1879–93.
32. Gameiro GH, Pereira-Neto JS, Magnani MB, et al. The influence of drugs and systemic factors on orthodontic tooth movement. J Clin Orthod. 2007;41:73–8; quiz 71.
33. Giunta D, Keller J, Nielsen FF, et al. Influence of indomethacin on bone turnover related to orthodontic tooth movement in miniature pigs. Am J Orthod Dentofacial Orthop. 1995;108:361–6.
34. Gkantidis N, Mistakidis I, Kouskoura T, et al. Effectiveness of non-conventional methods for accelerated orthodontic tooth movement: a systematic review and meta-analysis. J Dent. 2014;42:1300–19.
35. Goldie RS, King GJ. Root resorption and tooth movement in orthodontically treated, calcium-deficient, and lactating rats. Am J Orthod. 1984;85:424–30.
36. Gonzales C, Hotokezaka H, Matsuo K, et al. Effects of steroidal and nonsteroidal drugs on tooth movement and root resorption in the rat molar. Angle Orthod. 2009;79:715–26.
37. Gurton AU, Akin E, Sagdic D, et al. Effects of PGI2 and TxA2 analogs and inhibitors in orthodontic tooth movement. Angle Orthod. 2004;74:526–32.
38. Hammad SM, El-Hawary YM, El-Hawary AK. The use of different analgesics in orthodontic tooth movements. Angle Orthod. 2012;82:820–6.
39. Haruyama N, Igarashi K, Saeki S, et al. Estrous-cycle-dependent variation in orthodontic tooth movement. J Dent Res. 2002;81:406–10.
40. Hauber Gameiro G, Nouer DF, Pereira Neto JS, et al. Effects of short- and long-term celecoxib on orthodontic tooth movement. Angle Orthod. 2008;78:860–5.
41. Heckler AF, Mirzaei Z, Pereira I, et al. Development of a three-dimensional in vitro model system to study orthodontic tooth movement. Arch Oral Biol. 2013;58:1498–510.
42. Hirate Y, Yamaguchi M, Kasai K. Effects of relaxin on relapse and periodontal tissue remodeling after experimental tooth movement in rats. Connect Tissue Res. 2012;53:207–19.
43. Hla T, Neilson K. Human cyclooxygenase 2 cDNA. Proc Natl Acad Sci U S A. 1992;89:7384–8.
44. Hoogeveen EJ, Jansma J, Ren Y. Surgically facilitated orthodontic treatment: a systematic review. Am J Orthod Dentofacial Orthop. 2014;145:S51–64.
45. Igarashi K, Adachi H, Mitani H, et al. Inhibitory effect of the topical administration of a bisphosphonate (risedronate) on root resorption incident to orthodontic tooth movement in rats. J Dent Res. 1996;75:1644–9.
46. Isaacson JR. Your patients are on drugs. Angle Orthod. 2000;70:96.
47. Iwami-Morimoto Y, Yamaguchi K, Tanne K. Influence of dietary n-3 polyunsaturated fatty acid on experimental tooth movement in rats. Angle Orthod. 1999;69:365–71.

48. Kaback LA, Soung Do Y, Naik A, et al. Osterix/Sp7 regulates mesenchymal stem cell mediated endochondral ossification. J Cell Physiol. 2008;214:173–82.
49. Kaipatur NR, Wu Y, Adeeb S, et al. Impact of bisphosphonate drug burden in alveolar bone during orthodontic tooth movement in a rat model: a pilot study. Am J Orthod Dentofacial Orthop. 2013;144:557–67.
50. Kale S, Kocadereli I, Atilla P, et al. Comparison of the effects of 1,25 dihydroxycholecalciferol and prostaglandin E2 on orthodontic tooth movement. Am J Orthod Dentofacial Orthop. 2004;125:607–14.
51. Kalia S, Melsen B, Verna C. Tissue reaction to orthodontic tooth movement in acute and chronic corticosteroid treatment. Orthod Craniofac Res. 2004;7:26–34.
52. Karras JC, Miller JR, Hodges JS, et al. Effect of alendronate on orthodontic tooth movement in rats. Am J Orthod Dentofacial Orthop. 2009;136:843–7.
53. Kehoe MJ, Cohen SM, Zarrinnia K, et al. The effect of acetaminophen, ibuprofen, and misoprostol on prostaglandin E2 synthesis and the degree and rate of orthodontic tooth movement. Angle Orthod. 1996;66:339–49.
54. Kleber BM, Kogel A, Kogel J. Zur. The modification of the mechanically loaded periodontium during orthodontically induced tooth movement with nonsteroidal anti-inflammatory agents in an animal experiment. Fortschr Kieferorthop. 1991;52:204–11.
55. Knop LA, Shintcovsk RL, Retamoso LB, et al. Non-steroidal and steroidal anti-inflammatory use in the context of orthodontic movement. Eur J Orthod. 2012;34:531–5.
56. Kokkinos PP, Shaye R, Alam BS, et al. Dietary lipids, prostaglandin E2 levels, and tooth movement in alveolar bone of rats. Calcif Tissue Int. 1993;53:333–7.
57. Krieger E, D'hoedt B, Scheller H, et al. [Orthodontic treatment of patients medicated with bisphosphonates-a clinical case report]. J Orofac Orthop. 2013;74:28–39.
58. Krieger E, Jacobs C, Walter C, et al. Current state of orthodontic patients under bisphosphonate therapy. Head Face Med. 2013;9:10. doi: 10.1186/1746-160X-9-10.
59. Krishnan S, Pandian S, Kumar SA. Effect of bisphosphonates on orthodontic tooth movement-an update. J Clin Diagn Res. 2015;9:ZE01–5.
60. Krishnan V, Davidovitch Z. Cellular, molecular, and tissue-level reactions to orthodontic force. Am J Orthod Dentofacial Orthop. 2006;129:469 e461–432.
61. Krishnan V, Davidovitch Z. The effect of drugs on orthodontic tooth movement. Orthod Craniofac Res. 2006;9:163–71.
62. Landesberg R, Cozin M, Cremers S, et al. Inhibition of oral mucosal cell wound healing by bisphosphonates. J Oral Maxillofacial Surg. 2008;66:839–47.
63. Laudano OM, Cesolari JA, Esnarriaga J, et al. Gastrointestinal damage induced by celecoxib and rofecoxib in rats. Digest Dis Sci. 2001;46:779–84.
64. Leiker BJ, Nanda RS, Currier GF, et al. The effects of exogenous prostaglandins on orthodontic tooth movement in rats. Am J Orthod Dentofacial Orthop. 1995;108:380–8.
65. Li F, Li G, Hu H, et al. Effect of parathyroid hormone on experimental tooth movement in rats. Am J Orthod Dentofacial Orthop. 2013;144:523–32.
66. Liem AM, Hoogeveen EJ, Jansma J, et al. Surgically facilitated experimental movement of teeth: systematic review. Br J Oral Maxillofac Surg. 2015;53:491–506.
67. Liu L, Igarashi K, Haruyama N, et al. Effects of local administration of clodronate on orthodontic tooth movement and root resorption in rats. Eur J Orthod. 2004;26:469–73.
68. Lotwala RB, Greenlee GM, Ott SM, et al. Bisphosphonates as a risk factor for adverse orthodontic outcomes: a retrospective cohort study. Am J Orthod Dentofacial Orthop. 2012;142:625–634.e623.
69. Madan MS, Liu ZJ, Gu GM, et al. Effects of human relaxin on orthodontic tooth movement and periodontal ligaments in rats. Am J Orthod Dentofacial Orthop. 2007;131:8 e1–10.
70. Masella RS, Meister M. Current concepts in the biology of orthodontic tooth movement. Am J Orthod Dentofacial Orthop. 2006;129:458–68.
71. Meikle MC. The tissue, cellular, and molecular regulation of orthodontic tooth movement: 100 years after Carl Sandstedt. Eur J Orthod. 2006;28:221–40.
72. Midgett RJ, Shaye R, Fruge Jr JF. The effect of altered bone metabolism on orthodontic tooth movement. Am J Orthod. 1981;80:256–62.

73. Mohammed AH, Tatakis DN, Dziak R. Leukotrienes in orthodontic tooth movement. Am J Orthod Dentofacial Orthop. 1989;95:231–7.
74. Moura AP, Taddei SR, Queiroz-Junior CM, et al. The relevance of leukotrienes for bone resorption induced by mechanical loading. Bone. 2014;69:133–8.
75. Nastro E, Allegra A, Oteri G, et al. Avascular necrosis of bone in leukemia and osteonecrosis of jaw by bisphosphonates. J Oral Maxillofacial Surg. 2009;67:2701–3.
76. Olyaee P, Mirzakouchaki B, Ghajar K, et al. The effect of oral contraceptives on orthodontic tooth movement in rat. Med Oral Patol Oral Cir Bucal. 2013;18:e146–50.
77. Ong CK, Walsh LJ, Harbrow D, et al. Orthodontic tooth movement in the prednisolone-treated rat. Angle Orthod. 2000;70:118–25.
78. Pavlin D, Goldman ES, Gluhak-Heinrich J, et al. Orthodontically stressed periodontium of transgenic mouse as a model for studying mechanical response in bone: the effect on the number of osteoblasts. Clin Orthod Res. 2000;3:55–66.
79. Poosti M, Basafa M, Eslami N. Progesterone effects on experimental tooth movement in rabbits. J Calif Dent Assoc. 2009;37:483–6.
80. Potts JT, Gardella TJ. Progress, paradox, and potential: parathyroid hormone research over five decades. Ann N Y Acad Sci. 2007;1117:196–208.
81. Rashidpour M, Ahmad Akhoundi MS, Nik TH, et al. Effect of Tramadol (μ-opioid receptor agonist) on orthodontic tooth movements in a rat model. J Dentist (Tehran, Iran). 2012;9:83–9.
82. Rifkin BR, Tai HH. Elevated thromboxane B2 levels in periodontal disease. J Periodontal Res. 1981;16:194–8.
83. Rinchuse DJ, Rinchuse DJ, Sosovicka MF, et al. Orthodontic treatment of patients using bisphosphonates: a report of 2 cases. Am J Orthod Dentofacial Orthop. 2007;131:321–6.
84. Roche JJ, Cisneros GJ, Acs G. The effect of acetaminophen on tooth movement in rabbits. Angle Orthod. 1997;67:231–6.
85. Rodan GA, Martin TJ. Therapeutic approaches to bone diseases. Science (New York, NY). 2000;289:1508–14.
86. Russell RG. Pharmacological diversity among drugs that inhibit bone resorption. Curr Opin Pharmacol. 2015;22:115–30.
87. Sakuma Y, Li Z, Pilbeam CC, et al. Stimulation of cAMP production and cyclooxygenase-2 by prostaglandin E(2) and selective prostaglandin receptor agonists in murine osteoblastic cells. Bone. 2004;34:827–34.
88. Salazar M, Hernandes L, Ramos AL, et al. Effect of teriparatide on induced tooth displacement in ovariectomized rats: a histomorphometric analysis. Am J Orthod Dentofacial Orthop. 2011;139:e337–44.
89. Sandy JR, Harris M. Prostaglandins and tooth movement. Eur J Orthod. 1984;6:175–82.
90. Sari E, Olmez H, Gurton AU. Comparison of some effects of acetylsalicylic acid and rofecoxib during orthodontic tooth movement. Am J Orthod Dentofacial Orthop. 2004;125:310–5.
91. Schwartz JE. Ask us: some drugs affect tooth movement. Am J Orthod Dentofacial Orthop. 2005;127:644.
92. Seibert K, Zhang Y, Leahy K, et al. Pharmacological and biochemical demonstration of the role of cyclooxygenase 2 in inflammation and pain. Proc Natl Acad Sci U S A. 1994;91:12013–7.
93. Seifi M, Eslami B, Saffar AS. The effect of prostaglandin E2 and calcium gluconate on orthodontic tooth movement and root resorption in rats. Eur J Orthod. 2003;25:199–204.
94. Seifi M, Hamedi R, Khavandegar Z. The effect of thyroid hormone, prostaglandin E2, and calcium gluconate on orthodontic tooth movement and root resorption in rats. J Dent (Shiraz). 2015;16:35–42.
95. Sekhavat AR, Mousavizadeh K, Pakshir HR, et al. Effect of misoprostol, a prostaglandin E1 analog, on orthodontic tooth movement in rats. Am J Orthod Dentofacial Orthop. 2002;122:542–7.
96. Seto H, Aoki K, Kasugai S, et al. Trabecular bone turnover, bone marrow cell development, and gene expression of bone matrix proteins after low calcium feeding in rats. Bone. 1999;25:687–95.

97. Shetty N, Patil AK, Ganeshkar SV, et al. Comparison of the effects of ibuprofen and acetaminophen on PGE2 levels in the GCF during orthodontic tooth movement: a human study. Prog Orthod. 2013;14:6.
98. Shils ME. Modern nutrition in health and disease. Baltimore: Williams & Wilkins; 1999.
99. Shirazi M, Dehpour AR, Jafari F. The effect of thyroid hormone on orthodontic tooth movement in rats. J Clin Pediatr Dent. 1999;23:259–64.
100. Sirisoontorn I, Hotokezaka H, Hashimoto M, et al. Orthodontic tooth movement and root resorption in ovariectomized rats treated by systemic administration of zoledronic acid. Am J Orthod Dentofacial Orthop. 2012;141:563–73.
101. Sirisoontorn I, Hotokezaka H, Hashimoto M, et al. Tooth movement and root resorption; the effect of ovariectomy on orthodontic force application in rats. Angle Orthod. 2011;81:570–7.
102. Sodagar A, Etezadi T, Motahhary P, et al. The effect of celecoxib on orthodontic tooth movement and root resorption in rat. J Dentist (Tehran, Iran). 2013;10:303–11.
103. Soma S, Iwamoto M, Higuchi Y, et al. Effects of continuous infusion of PTH on experimental tooth movement in rats. J Bone Miner Res. 1999;14:546–54.
104. Soma S, Matsumoto S, Higuchi Y, et al. Local and chronic application of PTH accelerates tooth movement in rats. J Dent Res. 2000;79:1717–24.
105. Spielmann T, Wieslander L, Hefti AF. Acceleration of orthodontically induced tooth movement through the local application of prostaglandin (PGE1). Schweiz Monatsschr Zahnmed. 1989;99:162–5.
106. Stabile AC, Stuani MB, Leite-Panissi CR, et al. Effects of short-term acetaminophen and celecoxib treatment on orthodontic tooth movement and neuronal activation in rat. Brain Res Bull. 2009;79:396–401.
107. Suda T, Ueno Y, Fujii K, et al. Vitamin D and bone. J Cell Biochem. 2003;88:259–66.
108. Szalay EA. Bisphosphonate use in children with pediatric osteoporosis and other bone conditions. J Pediatr Rehabilitat Med. 2014;7:125–32.
109. Takano-Yamamoto T, Kawakami M, Yamashiro T. Effect of age on the rate of tooth movement in combination with local use of 1,25(OH)2D3 and mechanical force in the rat. J Dent Res. 1992;71:1487–92.
110. Tuncer Z, Polat-Ozsoy O, Demirbilek M, et al. Effects of various analgesics on the level of prostaglandin E2 during orthodontic tooth movement. Eur J Orthod. 2014;36:268–74.
111. Tyrovola JB, Spyropoulos MN. Effects of drugs and systemic factors on orthodontic treatment. Quintessence Int. 2001;32:365–71.
112. Vayda P, Loveless J, Miller R, Theroux K. The effect or short term analgesic usage on the rate of orthodontic tooth movement [abstract]. J Dent Res. 2000;79:614.
113. Venkataramana V, Chidambaram S, Reddy BV, et al. Impact of Bisphosphonate on Orthodontic tooth movement and osteoclastic count: An Animal Study. J Int Oral Health. 2014;6:1–8.
114. Verna C, Dalstra M, Melsen B. The rate and the type of orthodontic tooth movement is influenced by bone turnover in a rat model. Eur J Orthod. 2000;22:343–52.
115. Villarino ME, Lewicki M, Ubios AM. Bone response to orthodontic forces in diabetic Wistar rats. Am J Orthod Dentofacial Orthop. 2011;139:S76–82.
116. Wilson SS, Ayaz SI, Levy PD. Relaxin: a novel agent for the treatment of acute heart failure. Pharmacotherapy. 2015;35:315–27.
117. Wong A, Reynolds EC, West VC. The effect of acetylsalicylic acid on orthodontic tooth movement in the guinea pig. Am J Orthod Dentofacial Orthop. 1992;102:360–5.
118. Yamasaki K, Shibata Y, Fukuhara T. The effect of prostaglandins on experimental tooth movement in monkeys (Macaca fuscata). J Dent Res. 1982;61:1444–6.
119. Yamasaki K, Shibata Y, Imai S, et al. Clinical application of prostaglandin E1 (PGE1) upon orthodontic tooth movement. Am J Orthod. 1984;85:508–18.
120. Yamashiro T, Takano-Yamamoto T. Influences of ovariectomy on experimental tooth movement in the rat. J Dent Res. 2001;80:1858–61.

121. Zahrowski JJ. Bisphosphonate treatment: an orthodontic concern calling for a proactive approach. Am J Orthod Dentofacial Orthop. 2007;131:311–20.
122. Zahrowski JJ. Optimizing orthodontic treatment in patients taking bisphosphonates for osteoporosis. Am J Orthod Dentofacial Orthop. 2009;135:361–74.
123. Zhou D, Hughes B, King GJ. Histomorphometric and biochemical study of osteoclasts at orthodontic compression sites in the rat during indomethacin inhibition. Arch Oral Biol. 1997;42:717–26.

Index

B. Shroff (ed.), *Biology of Orthodontic Tooth Movement*,
DOI 10.1007/978-3-319-26609-1

The manufacturer's authorised representative in the EU is Springer Nature Customer Service Centre GmbH, Europaplatz 3, 69115 Heidelberg, Germany. If you have any concerns regarding our products, please contact ProductSafety@springernature.com

Printed and bound by CPI Group (UK) Ltd, Croydon, CR0 4YY

28/09/2026

02224078-0009